Advance Praise

"This is a story that needs to be told and Tom Glenn is the author to tell it. He is a skilled writer who uses his unique experience to tell a dual love story. One is the story of a straight man caring for a gay man dying of AIDS. There are scenes that will break your heart while they affirm that we humans are capable of profound love. The second love story is between a father and his daughter and the power of forgiveness. Glenn is a writer who can accomplish the greatest task of the art: he will take you to another world and keep you there and, in the end, you will know something and feel something you did not know or feel before you picked up this book. This is a book you will remember. Tom Glenn is a hell of a writer."

    —Larry Matthews, author of the Dave Haggard thriller
       series and *Take a Rifle from a Dead Man*

"In *No-Accounts*, Tom Glenn has created a small village inside a big city. It's peopled by ordinary folks who find themselves trapped in an era that gives no quarter, closed in with emotions that are always intense and always present. Everyone has to look grievous situations square in the face: how the shallowest selfishness has the direst consequences; how fear cuts to the bone; coping with love in all its variousness; stripping away prejudgments about "the other;" helping a total stranger go to his slow end; accepting one's own human mistakes and limitations; agonizing from wrongs wrought upon the people one loves and then trying desperately to forgive oneself. These men and women will get to you—you'll simultaneously condemn them out-of-hand, be utterly in awe of them, and hope you're fortunate enough to have their courage if you ever have the need. And Glenn does all this without a trace of mawkishness, weaving deep wisdom through the whole. Quite simply, it's awesome writing. Do yourself a huge favor—read *No-Accounts*. When you're finished, you'll know the human family almost better than your own."

—Grady Smith, author of *Blood Chit*

"Tom Glenn's *No-Accounts* is a novel of deep and meaningful compassion. Well-crafted prose and page-turning dialogue carry this story, but at the heart of it is sincere benevolence. In a world where charity often comes in quick, tax-deductible credit-card swipes, Tom Glenn reminds readers that reaching out and touching others in a personal way can be one of life's most enriching experiences."

—Eric D. Goodman, author of *Tracks*

"Tom Glenn lived his novel seven times as a volunteer assisting HIV infected men to die. This is fiction taken from life written by a hero who accompanied the terminally ill as far as any mortal could, devoting himself body and soul to their comfort and helping them make their exit with dignity. It is one man's story of committing unconditionally to another. A love story like no other, it is uplifting and wrenching and rewarding beyond measure."

—Juris Jurjevics, author of *The Trudeau Vector* and *Red Flags*

No-Accounts

For Ellen Kwrotnoski with affection and respect
Tom Glenn
17 July 2014

No-Accounts

Tom Glenn

Baltimore, Maryland
www.apprenticehouse.com

Printed in the United States of America

First Edition

Cover and Internal Design by Alexander Namin

Published by Apprentice House

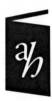

Apprentice House
Communication Department
Loyola University Maryland
4501 N. Charles Street
Baltimore, MD 21210
410.617.5265
410.617.2198 (fax)
www.ApprenticeHouse.com
info@ApprenticeHouse.com

Contents

Author's Note

Too many people have contributed to the writing of this book for me to acknowledge them all. The seeds of the story came from my years in the 1980s working with AIDS patients under the auspices of the Whitman-Walker Clinic in Washington, D.C. The clinic's training, support, and spirit made me understand the nature of the battle against AIDS and inspired me join in the effort. The manuscript went through intensive review in three different critique groups. I am especially grateful to Mary Eccles, a fine writer of children's books, and Ellen Kwatnoski, Author of *Still Life With Aftershocks*, a novel about the struggle of a woman to cope with the illness of her brother dying of AIDS. Su Patterson was of invaluable assistance in the final edit, and the staff and students of Apprentice House touched me with their sincerity, expertise, and hard work.

No-Accounts sprang from my horror at society's and the medical establishment's withdrawal from people dying of AIDS in the mid-1980s. Fear of the disease resulted in those who could have helped pulling back from patients; some men literally died on the street because family, friends, nurses, and doctors were terrified to touch them. I couldn't tolerate that, so with the consent of my wife, I volunteered to be a buddy, a sort of caretaker-*cum*-nurse to gay men with AIDS. At the time, we didn't know how AIDS was transmitted, so we had no idea of how much danger we were in. It didn't matter. The work was too important to let risk stand in the way.

We buddies did everything for our patients, even administering medications and giving injections, because there was no one else to do it. As the only straight man working with staff and volunteers in a gay clinic, my biases and stereotypes about homosexuality melted away as I watched the self-sacrifice and courage of gay men fighting a fatal disease. I went through seven patients in five years before I simply could not face yet another death. For a while I worked with the homeless and finally became a hospice volunteer. The searing experiences from those years of volunteering were the raw material from which the story of *No-Accounts* is drawn.

Dedication

This book is dedicated to the men and women who fought so hard to stem the AIDS epidemic. Their courage and determination permanently changed me.

Seek not to reward goodness,
For goodness is beyond reward.
—Hàn Hsīng

Part I

Dying Queer

Chapter 1

Male Bonding

Dying wouldn't be so awful if he could find Johnny's mother. He could almost see her through the gray twilight. She'd be tall and elegant and wise. He'd tell her the truth—that he'd known the risks and Johnny hadn't. He'd take full responsibility. She'd cry a little, thank him for his candor. She'd take him in her arms. Then the gnawing inside of him, like vermin chewing his entrails, would stop. For the first time in longer than he could remember, he'd be at ease. He'd face his father. *Nice goin', son. You done good.* Peter had done good? No, that wasn't right. Goodness is beyond reward.

And he'd be up front with Joey and Ron and Kirk and the whole crowd. Maybe even with Billy. Peter could see him through the fog, that fat-ass phony, fake from his ten-gallon hat and studded belt to the hand-tooled boots on heels that gave him an extra inch making him all of five-ten. Myopic eyes blinking behind contact lenses, paunch distending his flannel shirt, buck teeth shining red in the light of the neon over the bar. Now Billy was peering over the iron railing on the north side of the Calvert Street Bridge, staring down at Rock Creek Park. "If *I* was ever diagnosed, I'd boost myself over the edge and let go."

Peter opened his eyes. He was on the bathroom floor. Blood. He'd cut himself. If people came to help, they'd wear latex gloves.

His vision blurred again. He was weeping, drifting back into the colorless surf. Raising his head, he fought for consciousness and forced himself to sit up, but the more he lifted himself out of the haze, the more he hurt. The coughs and sobs were suffocating him. No one to call. Why couldn't it just be over? He pulled himself to his feet and clung to the towel rack, clutched the door frame, then the wall.

The bed was only a few feet away. He lurched across the floor and caught hold of the desk chair. His eyes rested on the desk. Where was that dog-vomit yellow brochure? That stuff about a helping hand. He eased himself into the chair and pawed through the stacks until he found it. "Charbonne Clinic of Washington, D.C." in broad letters across the top. Beneath was "A helping hand." He'd telephone the clinic. They'd send a buddy.

Martin looked at the brass number on the door and tried to control his breathing. Apartment 736, on the seventh floor of the Quebec Towers. His palms were sweating, and it wasn't the August heat.

He knocked. Nothing. He knocked again. Finally, a man called, "Yes?"

"My name is Martin James."

Silence.

"Peter, Mort Gray from the Charbonne Clinic sent me."

"Come on in."

Martin opened the door, stepped inside, and almost gagged on the raw smell of body odor, smoked cigarettes, and—he was sure—human waste. He was in the hall of an efficiency apartment. Ahead of him, the main room ended twenty-five feet away at a large, murky window, the only one in the room. Books, magazines, phonograph records, tape cassettes, socks, underwear, dishes, and papers covered the desk, the floor, the bureau, the top of the television, the yellow wing chair, and the small table in the dining alcove. Angry cigarette smoke hung in the air.

In a bed below the window lay a man in wrinkled pajamas and a stained bathrobe of the same royal blue as the bedspread and rug. The man turned on his side and glared at Martin. "I'm Peter Christopher."

Peter was dirty and unshaven. His hair was cold black, uncombed, too long, and shining with sweat, his eyes an unsettling blue. His face was a ruined sculpture with a classic nose, prominent cheekbones, hollow cheeks overgrown with stubble, and a sensuous mouth. What showed of his chest was darkened by hair.

The face, something about the face . . . With a jolt of surprise, Martin placed it—Michelangelo's *David*. The unformed shape of youth. But Peter's face had the shadows of an older man who had seen too much of life.

"Like to sit down?" Peter said.

Martin took off his jacket and searched for a place to put it. On a straight chair by a desk lay a telephone book, magazines, an ash tray, and a white tee shirt.

"Put that stuff anywhere," Peter said.

Martin moved the chair's contents to the desk and hung his jacket on the back.

Peter said, "I thought the clinic would send someone my age."

Martin tried to think of an appropriate response.

"You want coffee or anything?" Peter said. "You mind

making it?"

The tiny kitchen, adjoining the dining alcove, was littered with dirty dishes. The glass pot held half an inch of rancid coffee, and the plastic basket was full of moldy grounds. Martin washed the pot, the basket, and two cups, found a can of coffee, and started a fresh pot. He returned to the living room and sat by the bed. "It's brewing."

Peter rolled onto his back, scowled out the window, lit a cigarette. "Maybe we could start by getting to know each other."

"My name's Martin James. I teach music at Lincoln College. I published a book ten years ago—on Romantic Period use of the Neapolitan sixth. You like music?"

"Ever know a dancer who didn't?"

Martin fished in his jacket pocket for the intake file on Peter. "Says here you're a waiter and translator."

"That's what I told the aging queen who interviewed me. Mort. You know him?"

"Never actually met him."

Peter narrowed his eyes. "We all know each other. The gay community isn't that large."

Martin tried a smile. "I'm not gay, Peter."

Peter wrinkled his nose as though he had detected a bad smell. He put out his cigarette. "Didn't think they'd send a breeder."

"You want them to assign someone else?"

Peter shrugged. *"Tant pis, tant mieux."*

Martin said, "Should I go on?"

Peter nodded.

Martin cleared his throat and tried to calm his trembling. "I live in a rented house in Wheaton with three other guys," Martin said. "And let's see . . . fifty years old, divorced, have a daughter eighteen named Catherine. Most important person in my life."

"What's she like?"

"Too smart for her own good. Very articulate for her age—graduated from high school in June and will be starting college. Even got offered a scholarship at MIT, but I think she's going to turn it down."

"She live with you?"

"With her mother."

"If she's that important to you, why isn't she living with you? Why aren't you spending time with her instead of screwing around with dying fairies?"

Martin hesitated. "Don't get to see her very often."

"When did you see her last?"

"June."

"*June?* I thought she was important."

"Peter, we're not here to discuss my personal life."

"Yes, we are. If you're going to be my—" He signaled quotation marks with his fingers. "—buddy."

Martin glanced at the door. Maybe he should leave.

"Sorry," Peter said. "Guess I got a little nosey. Go on."

Martin collected his thoughts. "While I think of it—" He rummaged through his wallet. "—here's my address and phone number." He leaned a business card against the telephone. "Your turn."

"I told her highness Mort I'm a waiter because that's what I do for a living. I don't get enough translation work to count. I'm a dancer by profession. Before I got sick, I was really getting into Strauss and Mahler—even though you can't dance to their stuff. The way they use language—I did a masters in German." Peter took a drag and blew smoke through his nose. "Do you know *Der Rosenkavalier*? And *Das Lied von der Erde*? *Das Lied* is a German translation of Chinese poetry. After I listened to it, I found a wonderful book of Chinese writings. Ever hear of Hàn Hsīng? Then I lost interest and gave the book away."

He held his hand out, palm down, and studied his fingernails.

"For the record, I'm thirty-one and gay, and I work at the Nouveau Riche in Georgetown. Been trying to make it as a dancer for twelve years. Spent three in New York, but starvation was ruining my looks. So I moved back."

"You're from Washington?"

"Baltimore originally. My folks live there."

"You have a lover, Peter?"

Peter pulled his lips back from his teeth, but he wasn't smiling. "None of your fucking business."

"You don't have to tell me anything you don't want to."

"If you're going to be my buddy, you're supposed to know me, right?"

Martin tightened his jaw. "When were you diagnosed?"

"Eleven months ago. September 22, 1984, to be exact. That means I have a 15 percent chance of making it until the fall of eighty-six if you believe in statistics."

Martin had the feeling Peter was trying to shock him. "Do *you* believe in statistics?"

Peter raised his eyebrows, extended his hand, palm forward, and examined his fingernails. "Some days I do, some days I don't."

"I wouldn't pay too much attention to statistics if I were you."

"Don't patronize me," Peter spat.

Martin sat back as if slapped. "I had no intention . . . I'm sorry. I didn't mean to offend—"

Peter's eyes filled with tears. "I'm having one of my bad days."

Martin handed him a box of tissues.

"I'm really sorry," Peter said. "I don't know what's wrong with me today."

He turned on his side, raised his body with his arms, and eased his legs to the floor. "I'm going to the bathroom." Holding onto the bed with both hands, he shifted his weight forward onto his legs, stood upright, and let go of the bed. He was taller than Martin had realized—six-foot-two or three. He stood, as Michelangelo's *David* stood, with his weight on one leg, but Peter was leaner than *David*. His soiled bathrobe hung straight from his shoulders.

After a deep breath and a cough, he took a step and reeled. Martin stood, but Peter waved him off. "Get the coffee. I take mine black." He shuffled across the room. "Creamer and sugar in there somewhere." The bathroom door closed.

When Martin returned with coffee, Peter was on the edge of the bed. "Would you please prop the pillows so I can sit up?"

Wishing he'd remembered to bring latex gloves, Martin leaned the two sweat-stained pillows against the headboard. Peter wrapped his arms around Martin's neck. "Help me move." Despite the butterflies in his belly, Martin slid Peter's body to the head of the bed. At close range, Peter's stench was overpowering.

"Sorry I mouthed off," Peter said. "Let's pretend I didn't. Go on."

"How about if I clean up a little?"

Peter's eyes darted around the room. "I've been low on energy and sort of let things go. This place used to be beautiful. I decorated it myself. The carpet's such a deep blue, you feel like you're standing on the edge of a lagoon under a midnight sky. The dining room table and chairs are polished teak. And the wing chair—butter yellow. Matches the napkins and place mats."

In the kitchen, Martin found plastic garbage bags under the sink. He made his way back to the living room, picking up trash as he went.

Peter watched with a frown. "Talk to me while you work."

"Sure. You know who infected you?"

"I ever figure out who the bastard was, he's dead meat." Peter took a slug of coffee. "Why?"

"Maybe he's asymptomatic and doesn't even know he's infected. If we could locate him—"

"I hope the son-of-a-bitch is suffering beyond endurance."

Martin squatted to clean up an ashtray spill from under the wing chair. "What diseases have you had?"

"You already know. I told Mort all that stuff. It's on that form."

"Thought it would be a good idea for you to tell me about it."

"You a psychiatrist? What's with the pseudo-psycho lingo? I don't like being manipulated. I'm not a thing. Don't treat me like one."

Martin felt his face flush. "Sorry. Guess I'm trying to do it the way I learned in class."

"What class?"

"Thanatology. A class at the clinic to train us to help AIDS patients."

"At least you didn't say 'AIDS victims.' Or 'PWAs.' Christ, I hate it when people talk about me like that. I'm a person. I'm me. I'm Peter. I'm not a 'victim' or a 'person with AIDS' or . . ." he wrinkled his nose " . . . or a 'PWA.'" He took a fresh tissue and spat into it. "What does thanatology mean?"

Martin knelt by the bed and gathered used tissues. "Working with people with life-threatening diseases."

"Another fucking euphemism. You mean 'people who are dying'. *Dying*. Say it: 'dying.'"

Martin looked up.

"Say it," Peter said through his teeth.

"Dying."

"Thanatology means the study of death, doesn't it? Why don't you tell me that? You think I'm afraid to hear the words 'death' and 'dying'?"

"I'm sorry, Peter."

Peter threw his head back and laughed. "You, sir, are a klutz." He sipped his coffee. "In answer to your question, *pneumocystis carinii* pneumonia. The most recent attack was last Spring."

"What?"

"You asked about opportunistic diseases. I've had pneumocystis twice, plus the usual diarrhea, night sweats, weight loss, and swollen lymph nodes. Some thrush. No Kaposi's yet. Cross your fingers. No loss of mental acuity. No trouble remembering numbers and words. No coordination problems."

"If you had pneumocystis, you must have been pretty sick."

Peter nodded, his hand on his forehead, his little finger extended. "Very fucking sick."

"How come you didn't ask the clinic for help sooner?"

"I had someone staying with me."

Martin stood and emptied the ashtray. "A lover?"

"Guess so."

"Thought you didn't have a lover."

"Telling the truth is not my strong suit."

"How long were you in the hospital?"

"Three weeks." All at once, Peter's face turned serious. "I'm overdue to get sick again. I could die any time without warning. *Die*, Martin. It won't be a pretty death. What would you do if I suffocated in front of you? Would you panic? Are you scared?"

Martin clenched. "You scare me."

"Why are you doing this anyway?"

"Just want to count."

"What?"

"I want to matter," Martin said, "to do something important."

"Taking care of a queer with AIDS is important?"

"Don't you think so?"

Peter snorted. "One fucking guy who's going to die anyway? One out of hundreds of thousands?"

"Better than cursing the darkness, Peter."

"Better than teaching music?"

"Is dancing better than waiting on tables?"

Peter gave Martin a withering sneer and turned to the window. "My dream was to dance with American Ballet Theatre at the Kennedy Center."

Martin headed to the kitchen with dirty cups and glasses. He wet a dish rag and wiped the coffee table. "I wanted to compose. Haven't the talent."

"Maybe nobody ever believed in you or cared about you or encouraged you."

"Nope. Lack of talent. Anybody ever encourage you?"

"Had to make it on my own."

"Not even your folks?"

Peter grunted. "My parents? Shit, no. My mom—she lives in a world all her own. And my father—he thinks I'm the pits."

Martin gathered dirty underwear from the floor. "Because you're gay?"

"I've never told them."

"How do they think you got AIDS?"

"They don't know I have AIDS."

Martin blew air from his lungs. "What do they think you've got?"

"They, like, don't know I'm sick." Peter shrugged. "Don't see them much. Haven't been up to Baltimore since last year. They've only seen this place once. Two years ago. See, my father . . ." Peter scratched his crotch. "My father and I don't get along. He sort of wanted me to become a lawyer like him. He thinks being a dancer is sissy stuff. Actually, he's kind of a macho pig. Big on he-man swagger. Great out-of-doors man. Sour Teddy Roosevelt type. Very bully. Except when he's in his Grand Inquisitor mode. Most rigid Catholic I ever met. And Mom, she wants things to be nice. My father and I fight. We've had some real knock-down-drag-outs. So I mostly don't go home, and that makes Mom happier." He put his hand to his forehead again. His eyes misted. "I'm not usually like this. I'm much better than I was a week ago. Only I don't have any energy." He blew his nose. "You talk a while. Tell me about your love life."

Martin held up the underwear. "Where should I put these?"

"Clothes hamper in the closet."

Martin found it buried under a heap of sour-smelling, discolored pajamas and socks. "Don't have much of a love life. How about you?"

"Haven't had an erotic feeling in weeks. Makes me feel sort of useless." Peter tilted his head. "I can't feature you having a love life at all. You're a cross between Sigmund Freud and George Bernard Shaw. No, you're fatter than they were. Johannes

Brahms. Lecturing, yes. Making love, no."

"Wasn't always the professor type. Won't say I had looks to rival yours, but I did all right in my day."

"In your day? This isn't your day anymore? Is that why you volunteered to take care of fags dying of AIDS? And don't twit me about my looks."

"You're a handsome man."

"No," Peter said, "I'm not. Gorgeous, yes. Handsome, no. I'm not masculine enough to be handsome."

"Why do you say that?"

Peter extended his arm and inspected his fingernails. "Narcissism and self-pity, probably. Would you get more coffee?"

Martin filled their cups and turned his attention to the desk. "Should you be smoking?"

"Cohen—my doctor—recommended against it. He didn't forbid it. Like alcohol and sex. They all lead to shortened life expectancy." Peter giggled and coughed.

"You practice safe sex?"

Peter slid his body down into the bed and pulled the covers over his chest. "I think I've enjoyed about as much male bonding as I can stand. I don't want to offend you, Martin, but I really don't think this is going to work. In fact, if you wouldn't mind terribly, I'd appreciate it if you'd tell the clinic I don't need a buddy." He turned his head and looked at Martin. "I'm sure you understand."

Martin was too surprised to answer at once. "Sure," he said finally.

"I'm sorry, Martin."

"Nothing to be sorry for. Certainly no one's fault." He put on his jacket with unnecessary care. "They told us in class we shouldn't try to prolong a helping relationship where we weren't compatible with a patient." He was blithering. He hoped Peter hadn't noticed. "I'll call the clinic—"

"Martin, I really am sorry."

Martin shrugged and pursed his lips but couldn't think of anything to say. "Guess I'll be on my way. Thanks for the coffee. Sorry it didn't work out." He forced a smile and headed for the door.

❖ ❖ ❖

The next day was one of Peter's bad days, one of his *really* bad days. He lay staring at the colorless evening sky through the window and breathed carefully. He didn't want the day to be gone, not without something happening. That's what he hated most. Time, precious time, slipped from him and left no trace. No memories. No tracks. Nothing. Just gray. He used to be able to wait for tomorrow, when things would be better. Now he knew things wouldn't be better tomorrow.

His grip was loosening again. If he let go, he'd drift into the leaden twilight. His ass was sticky from seeping diarrhea. He needed to scrub the stink of rancid sweat from his skin. Hunger had gnawed at him for hours.

He sat up. Nausea flushed through him and urged him to lie down. Instead, he got to his feet. His legs trembled, but he didn't fall. He took a small step. Then another.

The sight of the kitchen stopped him. Filthy. He opened the refrigerator door. Most of the shelves were bare.

The room tilted. He clung to the refrigerator door and slid to his knees. A chunk of cheddar cheese was on the bottom shelf. He unwrapped it and took a bite. Another bite. His stomach reared. He vomited.

He sank back on his heels, closed his eyes, leaned forward,

and rested his head on the cold chrome of the refrigerator's rack. He was floating into the dream again. No pain. Only a widening abyss between himself and his body. The spindrift rising, gray foam and gray waves, shifting and flowing, turning, staying. He knew somewhere deep inside that he had to seize his consciousness and drag himself out of the swash.

But the waves embraced him, tugged at him, pulled back from him, rolled over him again. He opened his eyes and made himself focus. The cold was fear, not of death, but of feeling himself die. His body was sobbing and retching. He tried to lift himself with his arms. He couldn't.

He wouldn't live long if he stopped eating. Was he willing to lie in his own diarrhea and wait for death?

In the gloam, he saw Johnny's little-boy grin, heard Johnny's voice break as he laughed. Johnny's young body, so supple, so sexy. Could Peter die without doing anything to make up for the bad things? Was that what they meant by damnation?

Mopping his face with his hands, he took a deep breath and clutched the refrigerator door. Inch by inch he walked his hands up the door handle until he was upright, then staggered to the living room. The clinic. They had a hot line for emergencies. The dog-vomit brochure from the clinic wasn't on the desk. Martin must have put it away somewhere when he was cleaning. Next to the telephone, was Martin's business card. Jesus. He couldn't call Martin after yesterday. There was no one else to call.

He'll come. He has to come.

Martin sat at the kitchen table and sweated in the motionless air. The failed day was yielding to night. Remnants of the sun's sludge-colored light seeped through the grime on the window above the sink. The light touched the squat whiskey bottle on the counter, but it was too feeble to leave shadows.

He glanced at the green tile and once-white walls darkened by years of accumulated grease. He had tried hard not to find the house shabby, to see the little yard as casual rather than unkempt, and to judge his roommates as earthy rather than vulgar. He tried to keep busy. He read, listened to his stereo through headphones, worked on articles for musical journals, corrected his students' exercises. When the house was empty, he slipped into the living room and played a little Mozart on the piano—the one item granted him by the divorce decree. In the summer, he taught classes. In the winter, he took on extra counseling. In his search for contentment, he'd learned to shield himself from feelings of failure. He knew how to conjure an opiate to silence his mind when it had blundered too far into pain, to blank out his perceptions and blunt his instincts by submerging his consciousness in an unfeeling, endless sea. He could make his life become a detached dream. He could float.

Now, he was trying hard, too hard, to blur his mind. He glimpsed the bottle, closed his eyes, folded his arms on the table, and rested his head. He must not think, remember, or feel. Drift. Nothing but drift.

He could hear Vivien's voice cut through the air. Her earrings, large hoops, quivered as she spoke. "It's all over the office, Martin. My secretary talked to me privately. She'd heard about our 'problems' and wanted to help." Vivien flung her coat on the sofa and threw her briefcase and purse beside it. "Didn't say where she heard it. Best scandal we've had in years." She sat. "Tomorrow Arnie will ask me into his office. He'll explain he's heard rumors and wants to reassure me that he's on my side."

She was on her feet again. She paced. The earrings

shuddered.

"What colossal stupidity! A student! And bringing her into this house? Didn't you think the neighbors would notice?"

She raised her hands in trembling supplication to some lurking god, then dropped them to her sides. Her ears above the earrings were tomato red. "Take whatever you want. Get out. *Now.*"

"I thought we were going to talk it through—"

"Not after today. I want you as far away from me as possible. I want some tiny piece, some particle of self-respect." She looked at him without moving. "You demean me."

Martin snapped his eyes open, lifted his head from the table, and scanned the brown light through the window. He smeared the sweat on his face and the back of his neck. The bottle waited like a silent testament to his sins. Why did he allow himself to remember? It was four years ago.

Catherine had been only fourteen then, going through tiny rebellions to get her mother's attention. She'd taken to wearing Martin's old shirts. They billowed over her unwashed jeans, almost to her knees, like kaftans. Vivien threw a fit. She accused Catherine of dressing like a homeless harlot. What would the neighbors think? "Homeless harlot?" Catherine had said. "More like the hamlet hermit. You won't let me go anywhere. And you're home so little, they're not sure you still live here. Let's see . . . we're playing Alliterations. How about deserted denizen? Hapless hooligan? Motherless mutt?" Martin was secretly amused.

When he went to Catherine's room to break the news, she was on the floor, leaning against her bed, her knees pulled up to her chin, her body draped in one of Martin's castoffs. She wouldn't look at him as he talked.

"So Mom and I have decided we should live apart. I'll find a place to live . . ."

"Something I did?"

"Nothing you did."

She frowned. "Daddy, will you ever live here again?"

"Not anymore."

"It won't be the same. Not ever." She shook her head. "Daddy, will you ever come back for me?"

"I'll be back to see you every chance I get, as often as I can."

"Take me with you."

"Wait until I get settled, have some money . . ."

He hugged her before he left, but she sat passive, as if she were still trying to understand.

He should have taken her with him. She was lost to him the moment he said good-bye. He *had* abandoned her and deserved her punishment. By last winter, when Catherine stopped returning his calls, he had screwed up everything that mattered in his life. He himself no longer mattered to anyone. Then Johnny. In—what?—February?

Lanky, blond, and shy—a sweet kid with a constant grin and large hands that always got in his way. Martin was Johnny's faculty advisor, his mentor, his coach. Johnny was Martin's favorite. Never mind that they struggled over Johnny's wild harmonic writing and experiments in atonalism before he even knew how to write in the chorale style. Never mind that Johnny was now a graduate student and no longer in Martin's classes. Johnny was Johnny, and there was no one like him.

He sat in Martin's office, his eyes on the floor. The grin was gone.

Martin studied the black-and-blue on Johnny's nose and one

cheekbone. "What happened to your face? Were you in a brawl?"

"Doctor James, I need to change my course schedule. I need to speed things up. I have so little time."

"Only the rest of your life."

"I need to finish my studies within the year or stop now."

"Take your time and do it right, Johnny. What's the rush?"

"I have AIDS."

Shock stretched the skin of Martin's face. Fear shot through his intestines. His eyes darted to see where Johnny had touched his desk.

After that, Martin avoided Johnny. The papers said AIDS was probably spread through contact with body fluids, but no one knew for sure. In March, the campus newspaper printed his obituary—"Talented Young Composer Dead at 22." "Death from AIDS Sudden," the sub-head said. At the end of the article, Martin found the time and location of the funeral.

He stayed, ashamed and alone, in the back of the church, far from the mourners. He hadn't even tried to help Johnny. He'd been too frightened. He waited until the casket was gone and the crowd had dispersed, then made his way to the church steps and squinted into the spring sunshine.

"Friend of Johnny's?"

A small blond man in a tan overcoat stood next to him.

"He was my student," Martin said.

"I never met him," the blond man said. "I called and offered to help, but he wouldn't see me. I'm a volunteer for the Charbonne Clinic and the Hospice of Saint Anthony. We act as buddies for AIDS patients."

"Aren't you afraid of infection?"

"Of course, but somebody has to help. Some of these guys are too sick to earn a living. They get evicted and die on the street because everyone's afraid to get near them."

Martin's heart contracted. "At least you tried to help."

The man put his hand on Martin's shoulder. "You could help." He handed Martin an ochre card, put his hands into his coat pockets, and walked down the steps.

Martin raised his eyes to the window. The daylight was all but gone. He wiped his wet hands on his pants and remembered Peter's gorgeous face—not handsome, not masculine enough to be handsome—as Peter examined the ceiling and told Martin to leave. Peter was a real bastard. Martin was fortunate. He was free of Peter before becoming committed to him. Let some other volunteer suffer through Peter's unflagging, shameless, self-centered, flagrant nastiness.

I've really made a mess of it. His mind churned. He'd get drunk—again. He poured Scotch into the tumbler and chugalugged it. The Scotch burned on the way down. In a few minutes his consciousness would blur. He dumped more Scotch into the glass, guzzled it.

The phone rang. He jumped. The tumbler capsized, rolled, hit the floor. The phone rang again. It rang a third time. He wished it would stop. It went on ringing, every few seconds. *Goddammit!* He walked to the living room and answered it.

"Martin, this is Peter Christopher."

Martin couldn't think.

"I'm very sick," Peter said in a trembling voice. "Worse than before."

"I'm sorry. I—"

"I need help. Martin, will you help me? Right away? Tonight?"

Martin tried to make his brain work. "Peter, has something

happened? Are you okay?"

"Nothing ever happens."

Martin sucked air. As it flowed from his lungs, he nodded. "I'll come. Right away."

After he hung up, Martin walked to the kitchen. The tumbler lay in a pool of Scotch on the discolored linoleum. His stomach knotted. For a long time, he stood before the bottle. Finally he put it in the cupboard beneath the sink. He mopped up the spilled liquor, washed the sink and counter, and went to his room. He gargled with mouthwash, took his car keys, his wallet, and his oldest briefcase—packed before his first visit to Peter with latex gloves, denatured, alcohol, dry shampoo, incontinent pads, disinfectant—and left the house.

Chapter 2

Three Seconds

Martin parked behind the Quebec Towers on Porter Street and glanced at his watch. Almost nine.

He tapped at 736. Silence. He went in. No lights. The stench stopped him.

"Martin." Peter's voice.

"I'm here."

Martin dropped his briefcase on the chair by the desk and snapped on the lamp. Peter lay in the same damp pajamas.

"I was such a queen yesterday."

Martin's nostrils twitched. Most of the stink was coming from Peter himself. "Let me get you cleaned up." He turned toward his briefcase.

"Would you fix something to eat first? There isn't much."

"Let me take a look."

Martin turned on the floor lamp by the wing chair to make the room less ghostly. On the kitchen floor, in a pool of thick liquid, lay a half-eaten chunk of cheese. He sniffed. Vomit. He breathed through his mouth. The refrigerator was open. Yellow slime clung in strings to the chrome racks. He donned latex gloves and found half a loaf of bread on the second shelf. Moldy. The orange juice in a glass pitcher on the top shelf had separated. He closed the refrigerator. He'd get to it later. Prowling through the cabinets, he found a package of saltines, an unopened jar of pickles, and a box of salt. He went back to the living room. "Is there a grocery near here?"

"Safeway block and a half down Connecticut."

"What's your favorite dish?"

"Lobster with drawn butter. And a carton of Marlboros."

"Try again," Martin laughed. "Can't afford lobster."

"Hamburger patty on rice and a vegetable."

"Is there any rice anywhere? Any frozen vegetables?"

Peter shook his head.

"I'm going to the Safeway," Martin said.

He bought ground beef, frozen peas, and instant rice for tonight's dinner; eggs, bacon, bread, orange juice, milk, and coffee for Peter's breakfast; fresh carrots and apples for snacks; a room deodorant, bleach, germicide, and detergent. And a carton of Marlboros. He hurried back to the apartment. Peter hadn't moved.

While Martin was putting away the groceries, Peter called from the living room. "Hope you're going to fix something to eat."

"As soon as I clean up and make room to cook."

Martin refused to think about what he was facing. He put on fresh gloves and scrubbed vomit from the floor and refrigerator, cleared the sink and the stove, put water on to boil, and took the first load of garbage to the basement. When he came back, he poured rice into the boiling water, fried hamburger patties, and brought the peas to a boil.

As Peter sat in bed and wolfed down his dinner, Martin, praying Peter wouldn't throw up again, washed dishes in steaming water spiked with bleach, cleaned out the refrigerator, and scoured its walls and shelves. He used disinfectant on the floor and counter tops. The astringent vapors defeated the putrid odor. Martin's eyes watered, and his lungs smarted from the fumes. As he was finishing, Peter called from the living room.

"Martin, you mad at me?"

Martin stripped off the gloves. Poor Peter. Martin had been so intent on disinfecting that he'd barely spoken. He went to the living room. "No. Why?"

"You *look* mad."

Martin laughed. "Guess I do. So much to do all at once. Tell you what. You need a shave. I'll talk to you while I shave you."

"Better wear gloves."

Martin put on gloves, took off Peter's pajama top, laid him on his back, and shaved him. He'd never shaved another man. He learned as he went. Peter kept up a stream of chatter. "There's someone I want to visit. The mother of a friend of mine."

"Hold your face still."

"He died. I haven't seen her or anything."

"Stop talking."

"I don't even know where she lives."

"Zip it, Peter. I can't shave you when your face is moving."

Peter frowned but shut up.

"Open your mouth," Martin said. "Pull your chin way down. That's right." When he finished, he leaned back and folded his arms. "You look like a prince. Now we need to cut your hair."

"Don't you dare touch my hair."

"I won't, but you need a haircut."

"I'm too sick to go to a hair salon."

"Let's get you into the tub."

When Peter peeled off his wet pajamas and faltered into the bathroom, his naked body again brought memories of *David* to Martin's mind—except that Peter's bones were visible through his skin. He had little muscle left in his chest and arms. And unlike David, Peter's body was etched with hair. It started at the base of his throat and ran like a long, sculpted shadow to his toes.

Martin lathered and rinsed him, drained the water, and refilled the tub. For good measure, he added bath salts from the medicine chest and left Peter to soak while he carried the rank pajamas, towels, and sheets to the laundry in the basement.

By midnight, Peter was in a clean bed drinking coffee and watching "The Dance Theater of Harlem" on television. Most of the laundry was done, the dishes were washed, the worst part of the cleaning in the kitchen was finished, and Martin could walk through the living room without stepping in something. The place reeked of bleach and air freshener. Martin poured himself a cup of coffee and dropped into the desk chair next to Peter's bed.

"You're a good man, Charlie Brown," Peter said. "I'm ashamed."

"Why, for God's sake?"

"Because everything was such a mess. Including me."

"You didn't do it on purpose," Martin said.

"I made it worse than it had to be. I didn't call the clinic until I was desperate. Then I was embarrassed to call you after I acted like such a shit."

"Forget it."

Peter leaned forward. "There's a cigar box in the top right drawer of the desk. It's where I keep my money. How much is in it?"

In the box, Martin found a gold key, a hundred dollars in bills, a fistful of change, and an uncashed paycheck for seventy-eight dollars and forty-seven cents. "What are you living on, Peter?"

"I have a few weeks of sick pay left. Savings." He laughed with a bitterness that took Martin off-guard. "I was saving to buy a subscription to the Kennedy Center dance series. Take whatever you spent for groceries. Go ahead. I'm not a charity case. Yet."

"I didn't consult you about what I bought. Didn't pay much attention to what things cost. Besides, I ate dinner here."

"Let me pay for your dinner. How much did you spend?"

"About twenty dollars," Martin lied.

Peter grunted. "That was all?"

"I'd like to get you to the doctor, Peter."

Peter grimaced and shrugged.

"Want me to make the appointment?" Martin said.

"I'll do it."

Martin rose. "I'll be back in the morning to fix breakfast. Sleep late. You need the rest."

Peter's eyes were round. "I don't know how to thank you, Martin."

Martin checked him over one last time. He was clean and warm and fed, but his cheeks were concave, his blue eyes too large for his face. Martin put a hand on Peter's shoulder. "Good night, bunkie."

Peter smirked. "Bunkie, huh? Guess we're going to be on intimate terms after all. Want to crawl in?"

Martin withdrew his hand. "That's not what I meant. Old navy term. Means your workmate, your buddy, the guy who bunks next to you."

"I liked my version better."

"Night, Peter."

"Night, bunkie."

When Martin got home, the house was dark. He went to

the bathroom, poured peroxide over his hands, rinsed them with rubbing alcohol, and showered with germicidal soap. Exhausted, he set the clock for six and went to bed. As his mind drifted toward sleep, he saw Michelangelo's *David* with a sling over one shoulder. Uninvited, the tang of Scotch roused him. No. He'd ruled that out. Consciousness dissolved—he saw Catherine walking away from him. He called to her, but she kept moving until she disappeared.

Martin's team, made up of buddies for AIDS patients and a team leader, met each month at the Charbonne Clinic in a decaying row house in Adams-Morgan where there was never a place to park. The meetings cost Martin time he could have spent with Peter. The other dozen or so buddies on his team were gay; and although Martin was embarrassed to admit it, he felt uncomfortable in a whole room full of homosexuals. In fact, he hoped nobody he knew would see him going into a clinic known to serve gay men. Worst of all, the team leader invited buddies to vent. Martin didn't want to vent. The venting of other buddies made him squirm. Never mind. He *had* to attend.

So, on the second Wednesday of September, he showed up in the stuffy second-floor conference room just before eight. He listened to a series of announcements about upcoming events and endured a talk on the absolute necessity of using latex gloves. "We don't know for sure how the HIV virus is transmitted," the clinician counseled. "*Always* use gloves." Next came a lecture on T-4 helper cell count and an interminable graphic film on the diagnosis and treatment of the incurable and eventually fatal Kaposi's sarcoma—or KS as the other team members called it—a cancer of the vascular tissue in the skin and internal organs. The team leader's talk that week emphasized the need to expect the unexpected. "They're at death's door one day, ready to bar hop the next. That's how this disease works. We call it the Roller Coaster Effect." Martin paid dutiful attention as each buddy reported on his patient's progress. Mercifully, only one vented. Martin gave a terse run-down on Peter and his own emotional state. By nine-thirty, the meeting was over.

As he was standing to leave, the man on his left smiled at him. "Hi."

The man was an aging preppie, a small, lithe, blond guy with bright eyes, shining teeth, and—Martin checked to be sure—white shoes. All the man needed was a tennis racket. His face was familiar.

"I'm Mort," the preppie said. He extended his hand. "I did the intake on Peter."

Why didn't anybody use last names? Mort shook his hand— exactly like a straight man would have.

"We've met," Mort said. "At Johnny's funeral."

Of course.

"Feel like a cup of coffee or a beer or anything?" Mort asked.

Martin moved back. "Thanks, but I've got to get home."

"This your first case?"

Martin laughed. "I'm pretty new at this."

"It's going to get a lot rougher, you know."

"What?"

"Working with Peter. As they get worse, there's sweat, diarrhea, and mucus. And the endless baths. Then they get so sick, you think they won't make it through the night. The next day they rally. You never know what to expect. In the end, death wins." Mort lowered his eyes. "We're here to help each other. Give me a call if you want to talk. Here's my card."

"I'll be fine," Martin said.

"Keep the card in case."

"Thank you." He put the card in his breast pocket and left for Wheaton.

Driving to the Lincoln College campus the next day, Martin watched September descending in flecks and dabs on Rock Creek Park. The brisk air awoke an odd yearning in him, a longing without focus or target. He relaxed his mental grip and allowed the feeling to flow over him. Then he knew. The old ache. Like a festering ulcer. He was homesick. And he missed Catherine.

She lurked behind every thought. The smell of the air, the quizzical expression on the face of one of his students, the throaty laugh of the girl at the supermarket, a glimpse of his white dress shirts hanging in the closet—they all evoked Catherine's face. She'd be in her dorm by now. She'd be experiencing college classes for the first time. He could see her as she hurried about the campus in the fall sunshine, bought books that smelled of fresh print and new paper, met new people—strange people, odd people, exciting people. Was she still seeing that boy she mentioned, Albert or Allen or something? Martin wished he could ask her. He wished he could listen to her talk about her first semester at college. He wished he could just see her.

Never mind. Autumn had brought him comfort. It had brought him Peter.

The comfort went beyond doing good. He'd become attached to Peter. Peter's body—despite the ravages of AIDS— was so beautiful that looking at him was an aesthetic experience. And Peter was touching in his winsome feebleness. Martin's

feelings for Peter didn't stop there, though. Peter moved him.
Yes, Peter was a first class son-of-a-bitch, a spoiled brat, and a
prima donna. He also had insight—though he rarely used it.
He had a lost and pathetic quality, a waif-like aura, that Martin
couldn't fathom. Peter had something else, too—a sort of
indefinable goodness. Martin sensed it, though Peter kept that
part of himself carefully hidden.

Watching the trees and bushes on Porter Street from the
window by his bed, Peter saw the season change. He longed
for autumn's cool touch and the rose and orange on the maple
and oak leaves. The sky was the piercing blue that trumpeted
autumn's arrival. He remembered—smiling, his eyes closed—the
wind whistling on 42nd Street in New York.

Most of all he waited for his young blood to be stirred with
industry as it always was in the fall. He looked forward to the
swirls of energy he knew would charge his muscles, exhilarate
his mind, spark his soul, make him want to boogie. This year he
needed the recharging, the awakening that autumn brought.

Bit by bit, his strength was returning. He wasn't imagining
things. Martin saw it, too. Soon he'd be able to tell Martin
not to come every day. Maybe, with Martin's help, he could
even escape the apartment for a short outing. Maybe he could
snooker Martin into taking him to Cunniption's. Maybe Martin
could help him find Johnny's mother.

Maybe Peter would be the first to beat this disease.

His improvement was Martin's doing. For reasons Peter
couldn't imagine, Martin actually enjoyed working in the
apartment, shopping for groceries, and especially seeing to
Peter's physical needs. He took pride in shaving and bathing

Peter, swathing him in pajamas still warm from the dryer. Maybe Martin was gay and didn't know it.

Gay? Maybe not. Martin handled him with a strength, respect, and reverence he had never experienced from a man. Martin made him feel that his body had its own brand of sacredness. Martin believed that men always touched each other with respect—if they touched at all—as if all men were brothers. Peter shook his head. Martin was *so* naïve.

And yet, there was more to Martin. He had about him a sort of presence that attracted Peter. It was a kind of dull dignity, a boring nobility. Martin was slow-witted, bumbling, ridiculous, occasionally pathetic, certainly wimpy, sometimes genuinely sad. But before all else, Martin was a decent man. He treated Peter like a decent man. Martin thought all men were decent.

Peter surveyed the trees on Porter Street. The leaves would sport rose and orange soon. He smiled. Martin was a fool, but a good sort of fool.

◆　◆　◆

Martin understood perfectly well why Peter didn't want to see Doctor Cohen. The doctor couldn't do much for him right now, and he always had bad news. Martin insisted. Peter temporized. Martin glowered. Peter made excuses. Martin threatened to call Cohen himself. Finally, Peter made an appointment the last week in September.

Cohen's waiting room—white and chrome and smoked glass and shadowless, lit by hidden fluorescent tubes—could hold six patients if three of them shared the sofa shaped like a heap of accumulating snow. Martin sat in a nubby white chair next to Peter. He had never before seen Peter fully dressed. Peter wore black jeans and a cashmere sweater of royal blue. The clothes did little to conceal the angularity that sickness had visited on his body. His colorless complexion didn't help. And his thick black locks hung loose over his eyes, ears, and neck. He resembled a hippie somebody'd gussied up for a visit to a rich aunt. But no emaciation, no ungainliness, no lack of grooming could destroy the exquisite shape of his head.

Two young men Peter's age came in. They wore white sweatshirts, white denims, white sneakers. Clean-cut, wholesome, all-American. They sat next to each other on the sofa without speaking, glanced at Martin, ogled Peter, riffled through the magazines, twiddled.

"Mr. Christopher?" a woman's voice said.

The room was smaller after Peter had gone. Martin watched the two young men. He was sure they were lovers. Peter had told him that Cohen specialized in AIDS and related diseases. When the eyes of one of the men skimmed over Martin, he realized with a shock that they probably assumed he was Peter's lover.

Were gay men always better looking than straight men? No, they worked harder to make themselves attractive, and they spent more money on clothes and grooming. These two smelled just right, faintly musky, faintly sweet, a scent so unobtrusive that it hovered at the edge of awareness. The dark one had a Caesar haircut, combed forward, so that a wavelet of hair cast a shadow on his upper forehead. The blond's hair was barely long enough to lie down. Both were slim and muscular, skin faintly tanned and clear. Their matching sweatshirts and jeans were athletic in cut but snowy clean. Martin could imagine them perfecting their biceps and pecs before walls of mirrors at a trendy gym. He couldn't visualize them roughhousing in the mud with a football the way he had at their age. Might bruise or break something. Such solicitousness about their bodies somehow detracted from their handsomeness, made them seem not quite real, like fashion models. They lacked the innocence, the unawareness of self that young people shared with young animals. They knew how to show themselves off to the greatest advantage. That knowledge aged them.

Martin got to his feet and wandered toward the hall door. He browsed without interest through an offering of leaflets in a wall rack—the principles of safe sex, a listing of the symptoms of AIDS, information on the HTLV-III antibody test, and ways of fighting anal warts—all his, free for the asking.

Peter reappeared, flushed.

Martin turned. "What did he say?"

Peter moved past him and hurried down the hall to the men's room. Martin followed. He heard Peter inside a stall. More diarrhea.

The traffic on Connecticut Avenue made the drive home all creeps and stops.

"Tired?" Martin said.

Peter nodded, leaned his head on the backrest, and closed his eyes.

"Are you hurting?"

Peter shook his head.

"Hungry?"

Peter shook his head again without opening his eyes.

Martin let him be.

Back in the apartment, Martin put fresh sheets on Peter's bed while Peter soaked in a hot bath, then helped Peter into clean pajamas. He waited for Peter to tell him what Cohen had said. Peter was silent. Resigned, he told Peter he'd be back in the evening and left to teach his afternoon class.

Peter listened to the last echo of Martin's footsteps dwindle to nothing. He wanted to call Martin back. The silence of the apartment was marred only by the drone of the refrigerator, the hiss and hum of an occasional car on Porter Street, and the murmur of a television from the floor below.

Peter wept. He had steeled himself against regret. He had cultivated his cynicism and refused to look back or care about anything or anyone. Except the bastard who had infected him. No way to figure out which one it had been. There'd been too many. Half of them were dead now, anyway.

And yet, if he were honest with himself, he knew it wasn't hatred that made him cry. It was regret. Despite his smugness, despite all his defenses, despite the shell he had worked so hard to develop, he ached.

Sally had disappeared. Maybe she was dead by now. Billy. He'd hit Billy. He'd never see Billy again.

And Johnny, who never meant anything to him. Tall, blond, tan, and solid, more boy than man, with a silly grin. A good one-night stand. It had been in November only a month after Peter recovered from his first attack of pneumocystis. Johnny played the piano in The Back Door after the regular pianist left. A modern dissonant piece he'd written. Peter leaned across the keys, kissed him. "Can we go to your place?" "No. My mom. Yours?" "No." Peter took him to a hotel. "You believe in safe sex?" "Any reason I should?" "No regrets," they had laughed the following morning. Five months later, Johnny was admitted to the Hospice of Saint Anthony and died there.

Peter had known the risks. Johnny hadn't. Peter never told him. Peter never told anybody. Peter didn't care. If Johnny were alive, he'd go to him, tell him the truth. Maybe Johnny would forgive him and still this ache. Nothing could change it now.

Johnny was dead, as Peter soon would be. Peter could have spared Johnny, but Peter hadn't cared.

But, as far as Peter knew, Johnny's mother wasn't dead. She could forgive him, for herself and for Johnny, too. She probably lived in one of those Victorian houses in old Alexandria. She'd meet him at the door. She'd be tall and handsome and sad and wise, her hair gray at the temples, parted in the middle, pulled away from her face and caught at the back. She'd be wearing an understated long-waisted frock with a full skirt. He could hear her contralto voice saying, "So glad to meet you, Peter." They'd sit in the drawing room in front of a bay window looking out on a brick patio and seamless lawn. There'd be a fire in the fireplace. She'd serve him tea in a cup as fragile as a baby bird, so thin that he'd have to be careful not to crush it in his fingers. She'd wait, hands folded in her lap, head tilted, and listen to his story. He'd tell her the truth. Her eyes would shine. Maybe a tear would escape down her cheek. "Thank you for your honesty," she'd say. Maybe she'd even take him in her arms.

He had to find her. She could free him. He saw her stately figure, the tasteful drawing room, the patio, the fireplace. Around the edges of the image boomed the ashen surf. In his chest he felt the suffocation of pneumocystis. Terror of Kaposi's sarcoma flashed through his belly like quicksilver. The picture of his skeleton pressing against rotting skin blocked out Johnny's mother. Peter was dying. The end wouldn't come today or tomorrow, but as he listened to his body, he knew.

Shit, shit, shit. What was the use? He could pretend to himself that his predicament was touching, poignant, even gripping. He could conjure a scene with a wise and beautiful Mrs. Logan in a setting from Renoir. He was seeing his life as if from the audience. There was no audience. He was not Camille or Violetta or Mimì. He was head-to-head with death. No one was watching, brought to tears by the sadness of his plight. No one but himself. The heart-rending images wouldn't work anymore. Death was real and gritty and in-your-face. And there wasn't much time left.

When he pushed away the fantasies, what was left? Nothing but the steady trickle of his life, the leaking of precious time, the need to remember and try to repair the damage. To forgive and be forgiven. Never mind the fake Mrs. Logan. He had to find the real one. To do what he could to make up for Johnny's death.

Now it was Peter's turn. Cohen had as much as said so. He had told Peter that if he wanted to delay the next attack of the pneumonia, now overdue, he had to do everything he could to avoid exhaustion and unhealthy living. He *must* exercise fifteen minutes a day. And Cohen insisted that Peter stop smoking. Peter pushed back the covers, blew his nose, and lit a cigarette.

And of course, no alcohol. Or drugs.

"Every time you smoke or drink, you're shortening your life," Cohen had told him.

"Without all that—and sex, too—what's there to live for?"

Cohen shrugged.

"Then I don't want to live," Peter said.

"Are you talking suicide?"

Peter drew back. "I don't know."

Peter put down his cigarette and pulled the sheet and blanket up to his chin. *Was* he talking suicide? Like Billy?

The night Billy talked like that, the November moon was crumbling blue marble in an iridescent sky. A magic night. Only two months after Peter had been diagnosed—though nobody but Peter knew it. Kirk had picked him up in a cab at the Nouveau Riche at the end of his shift. They'd met Joey and

Billy and Ron at a new bar in Adams-Morgan, The Cock Pit. The four of them had ranged themselves around Peter at the corner of the bar where Peter could keep an eye on the action. All the talk was about who'd been diagnosed. Joey downed one too many shooters and puked. Kirk and Ron had taken him home. When the bar closed, Billy invited Peter back to his place on Connecticut Avenue to do some coke. As they walked down Calvert toward the park in the cold, piercing moonlight, the city around them was a medieval cityscape in a Disney film, blue and powdery and mysterious. Billy kept stumbling. Too much beer. Peter was drunk enough to feel daring. Right before the bridge, they pissed on the sidewalk, giggling. Then onto Calvert Street Bridge over Rock Creek Park, lost in a blue shadow far beneath them.

"You always see this bridge in movies about Washington," Billy said. "Maybe that's why there's so many suicides." He ambled onto the pavement from the sidewalk.

"Stay out of the street," Peter said. "Cars."

"No cars."

Peter looked both ways. He could hear the traffic from Columbia Road behind them and see an occasional headlight on Connecticut Avenue some blocks beyond the bridge, but no cars came their way.

"They always jump from the northern side," Billy said. He clopped across the pavement in his boots and stepped up on the sidewalk by the guard rail. "From the middle of the bridge." He stretched his arms over the thick top bar of the rail. "Right about here." He hoisted his weight, rested his chest across the railing, and stared down. "They're talking about putting up a fence to stop people from jumping."

Peter ran toward him. "Get down from there, you asshole."

Billy turned his face toward Peter. "Here I am all bent over, asshole in the air. Want some?"

"Billy, get down."

"My ass is too fat for you. You like bubble butts. Or all muscled up."

Billy's body shifted forward.

Peter tensed. "Will you please get down from there?"

Billy's face disappeared into the darkness, as his head ducked downward. "It'd be easy. Slide over the edge. Wouldn't be but three seconds before you hit. You'd never feel nothin'. Three seconds."

Billy's body slid. His feet came off the ground. Peter caught his breath.

"Boost myself over and let go."

In a panic, Peter grabbed Billy's studded cowboy belt and pulled. Billy rolled off the railing against Peter. They both fell backwards into the street, Billy on top of Peter.

Billy, his back on Peter's chest, spread his arms and legs wide. "Take it, man, take it."

Peter pushed him off, stood, and brushed his clothes. "Pig."

Billy laughed and staggered to his feet. "Scared you, didn't I? You thought I was going right over the edge."

"You're sick."

Billy chuckled. "I had you goin' that time."

"Come on. I'm cold."

Peter headed toward Connecticut Avenue in the middle of the bridge, following the yellow median line, as far from the rail as he could get. Billy skipped and stumbled along beside him, still guffawing.

"You're not funny," Peter said.

Billy's laughter dwindled and died. "Sorry, Peter. I was only kidding around."

"Don't kid with me like that."

"I said I was sorry."

They reached the end of the bridge in silence. Peter breathed easier. "We better get on the sidewalk before we get hit."

A block from Connecticut, Billy glanced sidelong at Peter. "I wasn't really kidding."

"What's that supposed to mean?"

"Just that . . . if I was ever diagnosed, I'd boost myself over the edge and let go."

"Come off it."

"I mean it. You ever see what AIDS does to someone?"

"Let's talk about something else."

"Okay, but I'd do it, Peter."

Peter stopped and took him by the shoulders. "What're you talking about? Neither one of us would do it. We'd keep having a ball right up until they carted us away. Man, we'd *boogie.*"

Billy nodded loosely. "Yeah, I know. We'd fuck until our cranks fell off." They began walking again, more slowly. "You never seen one of those guys. Jeez." He shook his head. "Peter, what are we going to do when we can't boogie anymore?"

Peter whisked a stray ash from the sheet, took a long drag on his cigarette, leaned back against the headboard, and let the smoke float from his lips. He hadn't boogied in a long time. Boost himself over the edge and let go? Three seconds until impact. Three seconds of terror, then nothing. His stomach felt cold. No, never. He wanted to live, as passionately as he could for as long as he could. He wanted life to be magic and rich, full of rose and orange, lilting and graceful. Not just lying here all day every day, fighting his way out of the gray miasma and waiting for something to happen.

He stumped out the cigarette. Maybe waiting was all there was left. How could he face another battle with pneumonia? His bowels glittered with panic. Suffocation. And yet he didn't want to die hooked to a respirator, a catheter stuck in him, all wired up, more lab rat than human being.

Or what if he got Kaposi's sarcoma? The lesions would shrivel his skin, turn it purple, brown, black, hideous. He'd hide from all human view, as Johnny had.

Peter'd found out about Johnny's KS one night in February, in The Long Shot. Kirk and Joey and Ron were there that night. And Billy.

And Eric. What a hunk. All bulges and fur in painted-on jeans and a torn tank top. Peter had seen him before and tried to strike up a conversation, but somehow Eric always escaped after a few opening lines. That night, Peter was determined. Eric sat there at the end of the bar cruising the scene, hunting for some ass. Peter tried to catch his eye.

Billy got in the way, as Billy always did. He was already a little drunk. He kept following Peter around and talking non-stop.

"Jesus," Billy was saying. He pushed his wild hair back from his face, squinted up at Peter, and blinked over his contact lenses. "Everybody's gettin' diagnosed. You know that cute bartender at The Wild Boar? The one with the beard? He's been diagnosed."

"Billy, let's talk about something else. This is depressing."

Billy nodded. "It is, real depressing. I found out a guy I met in The Back Door a few months back has KS. Real bad. They don't think he'll make it much longer. And he won't let nobody see him."

"Billy," Peter said, "that's enough. I don't want to hear any more."

"You don't know him anyways," Billy said with a wave and a belch. He rubbed his paunch through his cowboy shirt, rocked on his heels, and flapped his eyelids. "Sweet kid. Only twenty-two. Tall, with a big gawky smile. Johnny Logan—"

"What?"

"Sad case. Diagnosed a couple of weeks ago. You know him?"

Peter swallowed. "Never met him."

"They say Johnny's dying, Peter. Just diagnosed. And the Kaposi's is already killing him."

"*That's enough, goddammit!*"

Billy put his hand over Peter's. "Can I ask you something? What were you sick of when you were in the hospital? Level with me, Peter. Have you got it, too?"

"Fuck you."

Peter slid from his barstool and moved toward the hunk. He stood next to him for several minutes, then brushed against him, as if by accident.

"Sorry," Peter said with an engaging shrug.

"No problem." The hunk smiled, all teeth, like Burt Reynolds. "I'm Eric. I don't remember your—"

"Peter."

"Peter. Right. Peter."

"That's my name, not my most important feature."

Eric laughed. His teeth shone. Peter rested one foot on the rung of Eric's barstool. Eric leaned toward him, his eyes intent, exactly as Peter expected. What Eric lacked in verbal skills, he probably made up for in bed.

"You live close by?" Peter said.

Eric's eyes flashed. He was getting the message. "Close enough."

"What're you into?"

"Hi," said a voice from behind Peter's shoulder. It was Billy, beer mug in hand. "Mind if I join you?"

"Yes, actually," Peter said. "We're having a private conversation."

"Sorry," Billy said. "I know you guys don't want me interrupting or anything." He turned to Eric. "I sort of thought I ought to tell you that we all think maybe Peter . . ." He stopped and looked away, burped, blinked, and looked back. "I don't know how to say it exactly, but, uh, we all been talking and all, and, um, we think Peter has AIDS."

Peter's mouth dropped open.

"I thought I should tell you," Billy said, "so you could think twice, you know—"

Peter hit him in the face with all his strength. Billy staggered backwards and fell with a thud. His beer mug shattered beside him. The room was deathly quiet. Three men knelt beside him.

Peter examined his knuckle. "I'm bleeding. Do you have a handkerchief?" He held his fist in front of Eric's face.

Eric pulled his head aside and stepped backwards. "No— look, I . . ." He was edging away, slipping out of Peter's grasp. "Hey, listen," Eric said, "take it easy. Listen, I got to go anyway. It's late." He fumbled in his pockets and threw bills on the bar.

In the silence, Peter could feel all eyes on him. People were sidling back, moving away. *They know.*

"No!" Peter shouted, "let's *not* get together. Don't you leave. I was the one coming onto you. *I'll* leave. And for all I care you can fuck every queen in the place!"

Peter ran. Out of the bar, out to the street, out to the

darkness. Humiliated, raging, hurt. No regrets. No remorse. He'd wanted Eric. And he wasn't going to tell him. Goddam Billy.

Peter rolled onto his stomach and buried his face in his pillow. He hadn't seen Billy since that night. He hadn't seen Johnny, either. Johnny hid himself and died. At least Peter had escaped KS so far. He shuddered. *Please, God, no KS.*

He stopped. He was so changed from what he had been, but he was not so weak that he would abandon his atheism. What had become of him?

When he heard a key in the door, he realized that he'd been asleep. "Hi," he heard Martin say. He rolled over and opened his eyes. There stood Martin, grocery bags, mail, and keys in hand.

"What time is it?"

"Little past six," Martin said over his shoulder on his way to the kitchen. "Go back to sleep. I'll wake you for dinner. You really got tuckered out today."

Peter slid from the bed and shuffled to the bathroom. He checked his eyebrows in the mirror, pissed, and returned to bed. Lying on his back, his hands behind his head, he listened to Martin putting away groceries, drawing water for coffee, lighting the stove. Finally, Peter got out of bed and dragged a dining room chair to the door of the kitchen. "I'll sit here in the doorway so we can talk while you work."

"Sure." Martin frowned. "You need your robe."

"No, I don't, either."

Martin was past him and back again with the robe before Peter could protest further. "Put it on, grumpy."

Peter gave Martin the finger and put the robe on.

Martin went back into the kitchen and finished peeling

potatoes. "What did the doctor say?"

"My T-4 helper cell count is down."

"How low?"

"Seventy-one."

Martin grunted and put the potatoes in a pot of water.

"That's bad, isn't it?" Peter said.

"Is it?" Martin lit a burner with a match and put the pot on it. He stopped. His eyes met Peter's. "Yes, it's bad. I know it's bad, and so do you."

"What's a healthy count?" Peter asked.

"You know."

"Yep. Do you?"

"At least four hundred."

They eyed each other. Martin turned back to the counter and unwrapped chops. "These were on sale. Hope you like lamb."

"Fuck the lamb. I'm in the danger zone with a T-cell count that low. Martin . . . I'm going to die, you know."

Martin blinked at the chops as if trying to remember what he was doing. He took a frying pan from the cupboard.

"My weight's down to one-fifty," Peter said. "If I go below one twenty-five, I won't live long."

Martin put the chops into the frying pan, lit another burner, and slid the pan onto it.

"Cohen told me," Peter said. "I was suffering from malnutrition."

Martin stopped. "What?"

Peter nodded. "Before you started taking care of me."

"Weren't you eating?"

Peter shook his head.

"I thought," Martin said, "you had all these friends coming

in all the time to help you."

Peter shook his head again. "I lied. I was ashamed that everybody keeps staying away." He took a tissue from his robe pocket. "Where did you think they'd all gone since you started taking care of me?"

"Thought I shouldn't ask."

"I scare them shitless."

"You're the shadow they live in, day after day."

"Fucking cowards."

"Fucking cowards," Martin repeated with a nod.

"Why aren't you afraid?"

Martin lowered the heat under the chops. "I'm at no risk. I'm not gay, I'm not an IV user, no hemophilia, no blood transfusions, not Haitian."

"But we don't know for absolute certain that the virus can't be transmitted casually."

"Not likely according to the most recent research from NIH. They talked about it at the buddy meeting. High probability that it's bodily fluids."

"That's probability, not proof."

"Science *is* probability, Peter. We can't even prove that electricity exists."

"The point is," Peter said through his teeth, "that you know there's some possibility that you're risking your life by being here with me."

Martin peered at the chops. "Yes, I know."

"Other than me, you're home free. You don't smoke, you don't drink, you don't carry on with women. The model of wholesome, boring health."

Martin grinned. "I carry on with women every chance I get. I mostly don't get any chances." He slid the pancake turner under the meat and shook the pan.

"You could make chances. If you're alone, it's because you don't care enough to make the effort."

Martin's eyebrows went up. "Since when are you an expert on courting women?"

"I know, that's all. For instance, where is it written that you have to be here taking care of me and risking your life? If you spent the same amount of energy chasing skirts, you'd boogie. Shit, you'd have more nooky than you'd know what to do with. Why *are* you here, anyway?"

"Because you matter."

"*Matter?*" Peter snorted. "My parents are from the south. My mother was raised to lounge on the veranda and drink mint juleps while the darkies sang down by the levee. That's why she never did so good as a lawyer's wife in Baltimore. Anyway, she always talks about menfolk who aren't man enough to do *nothin'*. They're the kind that when they finish some work or other, you can't say, 'Nice goin'. You done good.' You don't say nothin' 'cause there's nothin' good to say. These men, they're no-accounts. They don't count for nothin'. They don't do nothin'. They *don't* matter. And when they die, nobody much notices." He coughed, took a drag on his cigarette. "I'm one of them, the no-accounts." He blew smoke at Martin. "That's why it don't matter what I do. That's why nobody much notices. People don't pay no attention to no-accounts."

"I notice," Martin said.

"You're a no-account, too, aren't you? You're a wimp, and you ain't got no balls. If you did, you wouldn't be here. You already said so. So it don't much matter if you care about me because you don't count for nothin' to begin with." Peter laughed.

Martin put down the pancake turner. "Let's say I don't amount to much. Let's say I'm a no-account. And a wimp, too. You're worthless and I'm worthless and I care about you and I want to look after you. We got one no-account caring for another no-account. Maybe that's all right."

Peter started to speak, then stopped.

"Get back in bed," Martin said. "You're getting tired out." Martin helped him to his feet, followed him back to the bed, and returned the dining room chair to its place. "Stay in bed while I finish dinner."

Martin watched Peter grow stronger, as if in defiance of Cohen's warning. By the second week in October, he was bathing himself. He asked Martin to come every other day.

"Wrap food in plastic and leave it in the refrigerator."

"Can you shave yourself?" Martin asked.

"No, but I'm strong enough for an outing. Will you take me to the park while the weather's still nice? How about today?"

"I have a buddy meeting tonight. How about Friday if it doesn't rain?"

Peter gave Martin his haughtiest sneer. "It wouldn't fucking *dare!*"

Friday morning, when Martin unlocked the apartment door, Peter was in the desk chair in loose jeans and a plaid shirt, grinning like a child.

"I'm ready," he announced as soon as Martin was in the door. "You?"

"Ready?"

"The park. Can we go right after breakfast?"

Martin smiled. "Sure."

Peter was too tall to fit easily through the door of Martin's VW Bug, but Martin finally wedged him in. He plunked the picnic basket and the army surplus blanket on Peter's lap and drove down Porter Street toward Rock Creek Park. At the creek, he turned left on Beach Drive and headed north. He parked, found a picnic table near the creek, and spread the blanket on the grass in the brisk October sunshine. Peter lay on his back, hands behind his head, and sighed.

"Don't lie in the sun." Martin said. "You'll burn. You weren't out all summer."

"I won't stay long." Peter glanced around. "I might take off my shirt. What do you think?"

Martin shrugged.

"I don't like it when people stare," Peter said.

"Worry wart."

Peter stripped off his shirt. His skin was so pale it was blue in the sunlight. The body hair on his chest and belly emphasized his protruding ribs. He caught Martin watching. "I look like something out of Auschwitz, don't I?"

"It's not that bad."

Peter arranged himself again, hands behind head, and closed his eyes. Martin rested in the grass next to him.

"Martin, you ever get horny?"

"No," Martin said, "I stay that way."

"What's it like?"

"Being horny? You don't know?"

"Being horny for a woman."

Martin surveyed him through half-closed eyes. "Level with me, Peter. You never leched after a woman?"

"Never did. I mean, they're pretty and cute and nice and all, but I never wanted to fuck one." He wrinkled his nose. "Doesn't seem natural. What's it like?"

"Don't know how to describe it."

"You think about a woman's body and you get excited?"

"Or how a woman feels when she's close to you. Or what a woman smells like."

"What do they smell like?"

"Come on, Peter."

"No, honestly, tell me. What's it like?"

"I don't know," Martin said, "they smell—I don't know—good. They all smell different." He relaxed and closed his eyes. "When they're aroused, sexually I mean, they change. Did you ever smell warm milk? It's sort of like that. Milk and honey, sometimes. Sweet. And rich. Like the smell of the earth in the spring." He opened his eyes and laughed. "I don't know."

Peter lay quiet for a moment. "Why did you leave your wife?"

"She threw me out. Found out I was having an affair."

"How come you were screwing around?"

"I really don't know why. Guess I was lonely and frustrated, and when Hedda offered, I accepted."

Peter raised his eyes to the sky. "What's it like to be a father, Martin?"

Martin shrugged. "You love in a whole new way."

"What's your daughter like?"

"Big girl. In heels she's almost as tall as I am. She'll have to keep an eye on her weight when she gets older."

"Blond?"

"Brunette. Her skin is on the pale side. She has hazel eyes. She can be quite attractive when she sets her mind to it."

"What's the trouble between you and her?"

"How'd you know about that?"

"You never see her. I got the idea you're mad at her or something."

"She doesn't want to see me."

Peter bit his lip. "I hope it works out for you. I hope she gets over it."

Was Peter being sarcastic? His face was serious, his blue eyes wide.

"Thank you," Martin said.

"I wish you'd talk to me about things. I'm a good listener. Maybe it would help."

Martin shrugged. "You've probably been in the sun long enough."

Peter huffed. Martin moved the blanket under a tree. Peter stretched out in the shade. In less than a minute, he was dozing.

The breeze shifted branches above them. Leaves, beautiful in death, swirled across the grass. The creek prattled out of sight. The air was rich with the smell of decay, the shadows long and hard, the sky a passionate blue. Autumn. The time of homesickness.

Chapter 3

God's Mistake

"What courses do I teach?" Martin answered Peter after breakfast the following Friday morning. "This fall two sections of elementary harmony and a sophomore survey of Romantic composers. Four of my harmony students have real talent. Three are incompetent. The other ten are average." Martin grimaced. "Best student I ever had died of AIDS. Bright guy. Great future. His death was a real shock. Got me to thinking about working with AIDS patients."

"Guess I'm indebted to him," Peter said.

"He drove me nuts." Martin gathered laundry. "He wanted to use the harmonic progressions of Stravinsky and Charles Ives. Not in my class. In my class, you learn to write like Bach."

Peter chuckled. "When I was studying at the Academy of Dance in New York, I was the same way. I couldn't understand why we had to learn the classical approach *first*. I stuck with it. Got to love it. I dreamt that someday I'd dance at the Kennedy Center. They didn't ask me to join the company. Not even the *corps de ballet*. I was crushed. So I tried out for every dance part on Broadway, off Broadway, and way off Broadway. Got a total of three chorus spots the whole time I was there. So I modeled for a while, but I couldn't make enough money to keep myself in cigarettes."

"You're handsome enough."

"Not rugged enough. Most of what I got was for gay magazines and shops. Then I worked as a translator for the New York branch of *Nürnberger Spielsachen* until they fired me for coming on to the stock boy. In '82, I came to Washington. A guy I was seeing lived here. I stayed with him while I hunted for temporary work until I could get a dance role somewhere. I landed at the Riche, and the money was good, so I settled down to have a good time."

"Sit at the desk while I change the bed."

"A little pot, a little coke, lots of booze." Peter flapped his hand on his outstretched arm. "I dressed in the latest and felt like I was *it*, honey, I mean, *it!* Had a different trick every night, several on weekends. Went to parties where we got into pot and coke and three-on-one and four-on-one scenes." Peter raised an eyebrow. "You know what I'm talking about? Sort of a *ménage à beaucoup*."

Martin tucked the blanket at the foot of the bed. "I get the general idea. But you did, um, *tricks*? You got paid?"

"That's breeder's speak. In the gay world, a trick is just a guy you have sex with."

"Oh."

Peter chuckled to himself. Poor Martin. He'd never understand the gay life. "Never mind, Martin. It's all beyond you. Anyway, it was getting *passé*. I got back into German poetry. You know Gerhardt Müller? I translated some of his unpublished stuff and the *German Literature Review* printed it. And I discovered Mahler and Strauss. Do you know the Mahler Ninth? I started working at the barre again."

Martin's hands stopped smoothing the bed.

"B-a-r-r-e," Peter said. "Where you do ballet calisthenics. Started writing poetry again. Hadn't done that since college.

One day I felt punk. Next thing you know I had night sweats and fever. I was terrified that I had AIDS, but there was no HTLV-III antibody test then, so I couldn't even find out if I'd been infected. Then I came down with *pneumocystis carinii*. You know the rest."

"You said something one time about a lover."

"Didn't amount to anything. I've never really lived with anybody."

"You can get in bed now."

Peter obeyed.

Martin pulled the covers over him. "Have you ever been in love?"

"Had a crush or two. Never really fell for anybody."

"You never loved *anybody?*"

Peter laughed. "Love's an illusion."

Martin said nothing.

"You've got a class to teach," Peter said.

Martin glanced at his watch. "Yep. Be back about six." He rolled down his sleeves, straightened his tie, and was gone.

The apartment was smaller after Martin left. Peter did his mandatory daily exercises—walking, squatting, bending—for fifteen minutes and dropped into bed, winded. As his breathing returned to its phlegmy normal, he braced himself for the boring day ahead. He was too tired to read, and nothing was on television this early. So he studied the ceiling until he had memorized every pock, then turned on his stomach. He decided to nap if he could.

Had he ever loved anybody? Sally had come closest. But she didn't count. She was a woman. Nanki-Poo, his Siamese cat? She—it turned out to be a she after he'd named her—had been devoted to him throughout his childhood. She died in his arms when he was in high school. Peter had loved Nanki-Poo. Anyone else?

The phone rang. Peter jumped. It hadn't rung in days. He lifted the receiver. The rasp told him who it was.

"Hi, Mom," he said, trying to sound pleased.

"Hello, darlin'. Hadn't heard from you for so long I'd begun to wonder if you'd run off and joined the circus or something." Cough. "I told your father you were probably working hard. And he said, 'Alicia, if we don't hear from Peter, it's because Peter is too busy having a good time to get in touch with us'—or something like that."

Peter rolled his eyes. *Sure. Probably more like, "That lazy no-good doesn't have time for us anymore. He's too busy wasting his life."*

"How are things in Baltimore?" Peter said.

"Same. Your Aunt Helen and Uncle Bud might be coming east for Christmas. They'd been wanting us to come out there, but your father can't ever get the time to take off."

"How is he?"

"Uncle Bud?"

"Dad."

"Fine, Peter. Why do you ask?"

"Wanted to know, that's all. Still working hard?"

"He'll never change. Tried to get him to go to Hochschild's with me to pick out drapery material, but he said he *had* to get ready for his hearing on Thursday, so I ended up going by myself, as usual. We're redoing the living room, did I tell you? I'm sick to death of that mauve sofa and chairs, and we can certainly *afford* better." She broke into a wheezy laugh. "So anyway, I picked out this lovely peach blossom pattern . . ."

Peter closed his eyes and listened. Would his speaking voice be in ruins, too, at her age if he went on smoking? Then he remembered. He'd never live to her age.

All at once, oddly, surprised at himself, he felt sorry for her. His father was as disappointed in her as he was in Peter. He hadn't shared a bedroom with her since Peter was a child. Had he ever been unfaithful? Peter was sure his mother never had. She'd done her best to piece together some kind of life for herself. She'd tried hard, with mixed and sometimes hilarious results, to overcome her southern country speech. Always dressed in the latest, though not always in the best taste, she knew what was in vogue in hair colors, moisturizers, eye liners, and skin toner. Carpets and draperies and upholstery took up her spare moments when she wasn't doing her "important work." Altar Guild at Saint Andrew's. Membership chairwoman of the Garden Club. Women's Civic League of Baltimore. Docent at the Poe House. Peter shrugged. She had her defenses. When things got too bad, she got very sweet and bleary and smelled faintly of gin and strongly of cologne.

His father's defense was his practice. Even when he was home, he stayed in his study, a room strictly forbidden to all, even the cleaning lady. He'd done better than his wife—his accent was pure Baltimore except when he lapsed on purpose. Traditional glum father. Peter couldn't remember what his father looked like when he smiled.

Peter scrunched his eyes. Maybe he could remember. He saw a young, bright face, midnight blue eyes, a five o'clock shadow, and a smile—large and broad, showing white, perfectly shaped teeth—like Peter's. A light slick of sweat on the unlined forehead, cheeks still flushed from a romp. Yes, it was his father in a different time. After a tickle fest. And then there was decorating the Christmas tree, maybe more than once. He saw his father switching off all the lights in the living room except for the little twinkly tree bulbs. He bent over until his face was close to Peter's, and he said, "Are you ready for the star, bruiser?" Peter clasped his hands and nodded quickly. His father put a silver star in Peter's hands. "Ready to fly like a plane?" Peter nodded again. "Turn around." His father slipped his huge hairy hands under Peter's armpits and lifted him, as if he weighed nothing, high in the air and set him on his shoulders. Peter recalled the scary feeling of his stomach pressed hard against the back of his father's head, his hands clinging to his father's massive forehead. The big hands slid down to Peter's waist and held him. "Go ahead," his father's voice said. Peter leaned toward the top of the tree. "Closer, Daddy." His father shuffled against the tree. Peter stretched until he could get the base of the ornament over the tip of the tree. He straightened the star. "Go around." Peter's father stepped first to one side of the tree, then the other. "Straight now?" said the voice from below. Since Peter was sure his father could see him, even when he wasn't looking at him, he nodded. His father scooted his arms back to Peter's armpits, flew him to the floor, and set him on his feet. Father and son stood hand-in-hand gazing up at the star in the soft light. "Looks good," Peter's father said. He stooped until his face was next to Peter's. "Nice goin', son. You done good."

Did that really happen? Peter wasn't sure. Why had his father changed into a wrinkled, misanthropic Mencken? That's the way he was in later Christmases when he came home and found Peter's mother drunk, burning dinner, breaking things. One of those Christmases, Peter found a half-empty bottle of gin behind the garbage pail under the sink. "So that's where Betty put it," his mother said, hands on hips. "Really. The help nowadays." They'd fired Betty. Peter fought off an impulse to cover his ears, as he had in those days when he lay in bed while his parents yelled at each other downstairs.

Much later, long after polite silence had iced over the quarrels, came the Christmas Peter would never forget, the Christmas Robbie died. Peter's cousin, two years older than him, Bud and Helen's only son, tall, lean, dark, sexy, funny. And *wild*. Stunning track athlete, football hero, the darling of his high school class, with a physique that made Peter's heart clench. Robbie had all the girls he ever wanted, while Peter, sickened at himself, wanted no girls at all. Robbie was the first man to make Peter hurt in that special way, knowing that he could never be Robbie, yet never possess him, either. At the beginning of Peter's senior year, Robbie rebelled, ran off, joined the Marines. He risked his life, not once but many times, the reports said. The last time, he'd volunteered to be pointman, to lead his squad on patrol through the jungles of Ca Mau. He was a hero again. There'd be a medal. Posthumously.

Peter was at the high school Christmas Ball the night the news came. In the dimly lit gym, all decorated with clear plastic three-dimensional stars and real pine trees and red tissue paper bells, he sat alone against the wall watching the dancers. The principal and two teachers found him, told him his father telephoned the school. He was to go right home. For reasons Peter didn't understand, his father had been enraged. Peter could still see him, pacing in the living room.

"Why are you so angry?" Peter asked, close to tears. "I didn't do *anything!*"

His father stopped, scowled at him, and said with steely softness, "You didn't do anything. And you ask why I'm angry?"

Peter had been rigid with terror without knowing why.

The following summer he sneaked into his father's study.

Over the desk, he found a framed plaque, with a quote from Teddy Roosevelt:

> Far better it is to dare mighty things, to win glorious
> triumphs, even though checkered by failure, than to take
> rank with those poor spirits who neither enjoy much nor
> suffer much, because they live in the gray twilight that
> knows not victory nor defeat.

He's ashamed of me. I'm a poor spirit. He liked Robbie better. Everybody loved Robbie. Robbie, who never felt the special hurt. Who got himself killed. Robbie dared mighty things.

"Well?" the gritty voice on the telephone said.

"What?"

"Peter, you sound extremely odd."

"Sorry, Mom. Ask me again."

"What I said was, will Tuesday evening be okay for us to drop by?"

Peter clutched. "Tuesday?"

"About seven."

Jesus. "I'd love to have you, Mom, but I'll be working. You know I work nights."

"You told us that the Riche is never open on Tuesdays."

Peter stalled. "Tuesdays?"

"Didn't you hear anything? Let me re-it-er-ate. Your father has to be in Washington Tuesday afternoon, and I'm planning to come along and shop for drapery fabrics at Sloan's. So we thought we'd drop by and see you after dinner, but if you're working, we'll come by the restaurant."

Panic flickered in Peter's belly. "Right, I'm not working. Of course. Tuesday. I was confused." He laughed. "Anyway," he said, feeling his way, "anyway, I haven't been to work for . . . three days, and I got mixed up."

"Vacation?"

"Sick."

"Sick?" Alarm rose in her voice.

"Don't *worry*," he said with a fast laugh, "I'm much better now. It was pretty serious, actually."

"What was it?"

"Pneumonia."

"*Pneu* . . . Why didn't you call me?"

"Mom, I knew I'd be over it in a jiffy."

"Peter," she said, "how could you be so thoughtless?"

"Hey, it was no big deal."

"You said it was serious."

He swallowed hard. "It wasn't fatal or anything."

"Promise me," she said, "*promise* me that if you *ever* get seriously ill again you'll call me. I'd better drive right down there."

"Mom, please. Look, the doctor says I should rest and not have a lot of company and excitement and all."

"Were you in the hospital?"

"No," he said, thinking fast, "no, I stayed here."

"Who's taking care of you?"

"I'm taking care of myself."

"Peter, you don't have the sense God gave a chigger."

"Mom," he said, "I'm fine now. I need rest."

"All right. I'll put off seeing you until Tuesday."

"Might be better if you waited until I was mended."

"Not a chance. I'm your mother, remember? And when a person's baby's sick, a person wants to go and see for herself how he's doin'. That's all they is to that. So you plan on us coming down Tuesday evening. Plan on it, now."

"Won't be up to entertaining much."

"'Course not. Wouldn't expect it. Nor would your father. And Peter, don't you go and pick a fight with him, now, you hear?"

"I never pick a fight. He always makes these outlandish, biased statements. I finally have to say something."

"He says the self-same thing about you, Peter."

Peter bit his tongue.

"It'll be wonderful to see you, darlin'," she said. "You take care, now."

"I will." He paused. "I love you, Mom."

"Why, Peter," she said, "thank you. I love you, too."

"And give Dad my love, will you?"

Silence.

"And he sends his," she said.

Sure he does.

Martin arrived before six and flashed his usual happy smile. "How are you tonight, mate?"

"Mate? Is that a proposition?"

Martin grimaced. "Navy talk. Don't read innuendos into my funny way of talking."

"Why not, sexy?" Peter threw back the covers. "Want to come join me?"

"Peter, that's not funny."

Peter laughed. "Not only a breeder but a prude. Guess that's the price I pay for not insisting on one of my own kind. Lighten up. I'm only kidding."

Martin rubbed his lips together as though thinking what to say. "You're acting like such a prick, you must feel better."

"That's the Martin I know and love. Yeah, I feel good. I'm on a roll."

Martin's face relaxed. "That's great." He headed into the kitchen. "I'll whump up a hearty meal. If you promise to stay in the next room during the testosterone storms."

Peter got out of bed, put on his robe, and followed. "No promises. *Chacun à son goût.* I'll be ready for another outing soon." He pulled up a chair.

Martin was filling the coffee pot with water. "Where do you want to go this time? The zoo? Great Falls? The Mall? Kennedy Center?"

Peter lowered his shoulders. "God, I'd love to go to the Kennedy Center." He tilted back his head and laughed. "We used to go there on New Year's Eve and waltz in the Grand Foyer. We got some serious frowns. One year Kirk went in drag—big white hoop skirt and lace and pearls and this foot-high white powdered wig, all curls and swags and silver bows. They threw us out. I used to have a party after midnight every New Year's. Champagne, balloons, serpentine, confetti, noise makers, hats. People used to talk about a 'Peter Christopher New Year's.' It was better than Halloween."

"Huh?"

"Halloween and New Year's are the big gay holidays, Martin."

"What about Christmas, Thanksgiving—"

"*Très bourgeoises.* Annual breeder coffee klatches. Bo-o-o-oring."

"I see."

"Liar."

Martin put bacon in the skillet and lit a burner. "Anyway, you think you're strong enough to go to the Kennedy Center?"

"Maybe someday." Peter let his eyes slide shut. He saw the

soaring marble planes and brass chandeliers and stairs carpeted in burgundy pile and tiers of shining white stone balconies. Uncluttered, massive, pure, masculine. "Do they let people be buried there?"

Martin sliced tomatoes. "Morbid humor doesn't become you."

"I mean it. Someday I have to decide where to be buried."

"I don't think they bury people there."

Peter cocked his head. "Actually, what I have in mind is Cunniption's. It's a bar."

Martin put down the knife.

"It's okay," Peter said. "It's a gay bar."

"And you want to be buried there?"

"That's where I want to go for my next outing."

Martin drew himself up to his full height. "And you want me to take you. To Cunnee—"

"Cunniption's. It's on P Street between Dupont Circle and the bridge. Kind of hard to park there, though."

"We're going to need to talk about your bar hopping tendencies. Feeling good enough to bathe yourself?"

Peter nodded.

"Go take your shower," Martin said, "then we'll talk while we eat. I'm going to get the soup going and take a load of laundry down."

"And I need a haircut, too."

At dinner, Peter finished his BLT and mushroom soup—he didn't even mention that he hated mushroom soup—and asked for dessert.

Martin looked at him sidelong. "Trying to impress me?"

"Trying not to lose any more weight. Maybe I could even gain a pound or two."

"Great. I'll dish you out some ice cream."

"With chocolate sauce and whipped cream, please."

Martin started for the kitchen, then stopped. "Why do I feel like I'm being set up?"

"My parents are coming to visit Tuesday night. Butter pecan."

Martin jumped. "What?"

"Butter pecan. Not chocolate swirl. Chocolate swirl is *not* good with chocolate sauce."

"Your parents are coming?"

"Martin, get the ice cream, then I'll tell you the whole thing."

Martin scooped. He carried the bowl—butter pecan, chocolate sauce, whipped cream over the whole thing—back to the dining room table and put it down in front of Peter.

"And coffee."

"Peter—"

Martin growled, poured coffee, and plunked down opposite Peter.

Peter told him about his mother's call. "That reminds me. Dad drinks Scotch, and Mom drinks gin. We'll have to buy booze."

"'We?'"

"Hope you'll be here, Martin."

"If you want me. Guess it's going to be rough. They haven't seen you since you started losing weight? Oh, boy." Martin clucked his tongue and shook his head. "Thought about how you're going to tell them? Want to practice with me or anything?"

"I'm not going to tell them."

Martin blinked. "I mean about AIDS. And being gay."

"I'm not going to tell them, Martin."

"Peter, what are you talking about? One look at you and they'll know."

"Know what? I told my mom I had pneumonia, and that it was bad, and so she's expecting me to be puny."

Martin put his hand on Peter's shoulder. "Peter, my friend, you're worse than puny."

"I don't care, Martin. I don't want them to know. I couldn't stop them from coming, but I'll fool them somehow."

"Why?" Martin said. "Why don't you just tell them?"

"Because they'd never forgive me."

"*Forgive* you? Peter—"

"They wouldn't, Martin. I know. Will you help me?"

"God. I don't know. This is serious."

"Please. I can't do it by myself."

Martin took a deep breath and nodded. "Yeah, okay. Jesus."

Peter sighed and sat back. He was drained. He nodded at his untouched ice cream and fluttered his eyes at Martin. "I can't finish my ice cream. Be an angel and save it for me?"

Over the weekend, Martin watched as Peter searched though his clothes for the best combination to conceal his thinness. He tried on outfit after outfit. He ate as much as he could stand. Tuesday morning, he gave Martin money to buy liquor on the way back from morning classes. Martin returned in the middle of the day with the gin, Scotch, mixes, and a bundle of yellow and white carnations. Then he was off to teach his two o'clock and hold office hours.

At five-twenty, Martin was back, breathless. Inside the door he stopped dead. The bed was made, set up as a sort of sofa with bolsters. The flowers stood like a frozen sunburst at the center of the table in the alcove surrounded by liquor decanters, glasses, an ice bucket, tongs, and three symmetrical stacks of small blue-and-yellow paper napkins—as if for a full-fledged cocktail party. Peter was in the yellow wing chair fully dressed in a white turtleneck, a loose fitting wine-colored cardigan buttoned at the navel, and royal blue slacks. His hair was combed back. His face was fuller than Martin had ever seen it. Peter almost looked fat. Martin switched on the desk light and gaped at him.

"Turn the light off," Peter snapped.

"What have you done to yourself?"

"What do you think? Will they be able to tell?"

"You look healthier than I've ever seen you. Fess up."

"Stuffing," Peter whispered. "See?" He lifted his shirt and showed Martin the wadding inside. "And make-up. I told you I studied at the Academy. One of the things a dancer knows is make-up. I spent most of the afternoon on it. Does it show?"

"No. I can't believe it."

"Now, two things are very important. The first is that nobody turn on too many lights. And second, I don't want them to get any closer to me than they absolutely have to."

"Won't your mother want to hug you?"

"I thought of that. I'm going to tell her I'm still infectious."

"God, you're amazing."

"Think it'll work?"

Throughout dinner and dishes, Peter reviewed every detail of the plot. While Martin dry-mopped the kitchen floor, Peter filled the ice bucket, turned off the lights except the lamp on the desk, the floor lamp behind the wing chair, and the overhead bulb in the kitchen. He put the soundtrack from *Breakfast at Tiffany's* on the stereo, lowered the volume, and went to the bathroom. By six-forty-five, he was lolling in the wing chair, cigarette drooping from his outstretched fingers, his face a mask of insouciant laze.

"Martin, put your coat and tie on."

Martin tied his tie in front of the mirror in the hall. "Aren't you tired?"

"Exhausted." Peter grinned. "Get me a drink. And get yourself one, so they'll think we've been lounging around sloshing a few."

"You're enjoying this."

"See the decanter with the metal tag on it that says 'Scotch'?"

Martin's stomach shifted. Of all drinks, why did it have to be Scotch?

"It's not Scotch," Peter said. "It's tea. Serve me that. The real Scotch is in the other bottle."

Martin poured the tea over ice cubes.

"That's another trick I learned in New York," Peter said. "Cold tea looks exactly like booze. On stage—"

A knock. Peter put his index finger to his lips and checked the room once more. Another knock. Peter lounged back, lit a fresh cigarette, and crossed his legs. He tipped his head toward the door. Martin opened it.

In the hall stood a ruddy frowning man in a navy pinstripe three-piece suit and a stocky woman in a black crepe pantsuit, three-inch heels, and shoulder length, black, Dolly Parton hair. The man was Martin's age and size, but he was in better shape and had far less hair and no beard. He stood erect, like a man used to depending on his body, a woodsman or athlete. His eyes caught Martin's attention. Sadness congealed into hostility as he watched Martin's face.

The woman seemed too young to be Peter's mother. No gray

in her rigid hair, no lines visible in her carefully made-up face. She wore a crystal pendant with matching earrings, dangling transparent spheres, that swung as she moved her head to peer past Martin into the darkened apartment. When she put her hands to her mouth, Martin saw that they were veined and wrinkled. "I'm terribly sorry," she said in a drawl. She stepped back, wrinkled her brow, and squinted at the number on the door. "We were trying to find 736."

"This is it," Martin said. "Mr. and Mrs. Christopher?" He opened the door wide and stepped back.

The woman gave him an exaggerated smile, all teeth between stretched, glossed lips, and moved uncertainly into the apartment, the man at her elbow. They peeped into the half-light.

"Peter," the woman cried.

"Hold it, Mom." Peter thrust the palm of his hand toward her. "I'm still infectious. Better not come too close. Mom, Dad, Martin James."

"Alicia and Roger," she said. "How do you do, Mr. James?"

"It's Doctor James, mother," Peter said.

Alicia appraised Martin. "You're Peter's doctor?"

"No, no. A friend."

"Goodness," Alicia said. "Peter's moving up in the world."

"Not really," Martin laughed. "I'm not a physician. College professor. Call me Martin."

Alicia frowned as though she sensed something awry.

"Sit down, everyone," Peter said with sudden graciousness. "I hope you'll excuse me for staying put, but I'm 'bout wore out." He laughed and put out his cigarette. "The doctor told me to take it easy, but Martin and I did a couple of sets of tennis. One probably would have been enough."

Martin gawked at him. He gave Martin a fatuous smile.

"You're out playing tennis and you're still infectious?" Alicia said.

Martin tightened his jaw and pulled up chairs from the desk and dining alcove.

"Ain't that the damnedest thing?" Peter said. "Actually, except for being a little weak, I'm completely over being sick, but I can't go back to work yet. Board of Health would have a fit."

"I thought you told me you had pneumonia." Alicia fumbled in her purse, pulled out a filigreed cigarette case and a jeweled lighter. "And since when is pneumonia infectious?"

"Some kinds are. What I have is. Viral pneumonia. Ask Martin."

Martin could have slugged him. "Certainly. Yes. Viral, you know, it's really bad stuff. You don't see me going near him." Martin joined in the polite laughter.

"What're you drinking?" Peter sparkled. He leaned forward, his arms folded on his knees. "Martin, would you mind doing the honors? Don't want to spread my germs."

Martin felt more and more like a player in a late afternoon rerun. "What'll it be?"

"Gin and tonic," Alicia said, "and double the gin. Been a long day, and I'm drier than a dromedary during drought."

Roger winced. "Scotch and water."

"And I'll have another Scotch," Peter said.

Martin mixed and served. He made sure he didn't confuse the two bottles of Scotch. The aroma of the real Scotch made him gag.

"Now," Alicia said, settling back in her chair, "tell me about this . . ." She wrinkled her nose. " . . . pneumonia."

"Not much to tell," Peter said with a short laugh. "Mild

case. Walking viral pneumonia. Got over it quick, but it takes the starch out of you. I'll need a few days to get the old heave-ho back."

"How'd you get it?" Roger said.

"Damned if I know. I hear it's been going around."

"That's the trouble with D.C.," Alicia said. "So unhealthy. It attracts undesirable elements. Like New York City, but . . ." She scrabbled in her purse. "It does have the loveliest stores." She brandished a clutch of drapery, carpet, and upholstery samples.

"Nice," Peter said.

She giggled and put her hand to her throat. "Guess I'm in my peach and coral period. You know, like Picasso's blue period?" Giggle. "Anyway, that paler set, the more pastel pieces, on the bottom, they're from Hochschild's. The dustier ones are Sloan's. What do you think?"

Peter shrugged. "I'd have to see them in the room."

She nodded once. "That's what I told that girl. Pushy little thing. A Negra with too much make-up and some kind of awful cologne. She was all for having me sign a contract for them to come out. Introduced me to their 'designer.' This prissy young fellow, all lisp and limp wrist." She shook her head sadly. "In my day, those people never could have worked in one of the *good* stores."

Peter turned to Roger. "What brought you to D.C.?"

"I *think* I like the darker set better," Alicia said. "More subtle, more mature."

"Consultation," Roger said. "I'm defending a company being sued by a guy they fired—"

"More in keeping with the understated elegance of the house," Alicia said. "Don't you think?"

"He got AIDS and the company let him go," Roger said.

Peter froze in mid-sip.

"I asked you a question," Alicia said.

"Sorry," Peter said. "What?"

"Oh, never mind." She put her glass down with a clunk. "Don't know why I bothered." She stuffed the samples back into her purse.

"Like I said, I'd have to see them in the setting," Peter said. "AIDS?"

"Why go to all the trouble," Alicia said, "when nobody's going to even notice? You'll probably never trouble yourself to come out and see it when it's done."

"It's contagious," Roger said.

"When *are* you going to find time to visit your parents?" Alicia said.

"Not from casual contact," Peter said.

"Peter!" Alicia said. "I'm speaking to you. Remember me? Your mother?"

Peter rubbed the back of his neck as though it hurt. "Sorry. How about Thanksgiving?"

"I won't have the redecorating finished."

"Then I won't come," Peter said with a smirk.

"Don't be a smart aleck," she said.

"Where did you and Peter meet?" Roger said to Martin. Martin bumbled.

"New York," Peter said. "Martin's a composer. He was working on a score to a new ballet I tried out for. We have a lot in common."

Alicia looked from one to the other. "Really?"

"Are you married, Martin?" Roger asked.

"Divorced." Martin sipped his tea.

"I'm sorry," Roger said, not sorry at all.

"Oh . . ." Martin waved his hand and wondered what he was supposed to say.

"Children?" Alicia asked.

"One daughter," Martin said. "Starting at The George Washington University."

"Do tell her to be careful," Alicia said. "There's so many— what shall I call them?—undesirable elements at GW." She tipped back her head and laughed. "I don't mean to be biased. It's not that, but you *do* have to be careful nowadays."

"Come on, Mom," Peter said. "Undesirable elements?"

"*Peter*," she said with a teasing smile. "You *know* what I mean. All those foreign students. Arabs, and Iranians, and God only knows what. And the blacks, for heaven's sake. And those *gays*." She sipped again and shook her head, still swallowing. "I know you don't agree with me, Peter, but those people don't live by the same rules as folks like us. They just don't, now." She nodded resolutely to underscore her words.

Martin tensed. Peter's grin wilted.

Alicia fluttered her hands. "Tell your daughter to steer clear of the undesirable elements."

All four sipped.

"Aunt Helen and Uncle Bud might be coming for Christmas?" Peter said.

Roger said, "They haven't decided."

"Do they ever . . ." Peter stopped as though he couldn't decide what to say. "Ever talk about Robbie?"

"Never mention him," Roger said, "but they've never really been the same. Every December seventeenth . . ." He shook his head.

"I told Helen at the time," Alicia said, "that it was best to get past it. Should have saved my breath. That boy. Always taking chances. 'Course, I never said anything to Helen, but he had no one but himself to blame."

"Lay off Robbie, Alicia," Roger said. "He was a fine young man."

"You still grieve over him?" Peter said.

"Robbie?" Roger laughed. "That was years ago."

"You were close to him."

"He wasn't *my* son. I feel bad for Bud sometimes. Robbie had so much promise. Bud was so proud of him. Spoiled him rotten. Robbie could do no wrong. When he was a baby, I used to kid Bud that he should have named him Emmanuel Christopher."

"He dared mighty things," Peter said.

Roger gave Peter a questioning look.

"Tell me more," Peter said, "about the AIDS case."

"They let him go," Alicia said, "and he screamed prejudice— *prejudice*, can you imagine?—and sued."

Martin grazed Peter with his eyes.

"It's not settled yet," Roger said. "Frankly, we're waiting for him to die or get so sick he'll quit making a fuss."

Martin closed his eyes.

"I know that sounds heartless," Roger continued, "but he did bring it on himself, after all, by engaging in certain acts better left unspecified. There's no reason why others should have to suffer because of his personal history. And the law isn't equipped to handle the situation."

"Why did they fire him?" Peter asked.

"Christ, anybody could get it from him," Roger said. "You can't have people like that working with normal folks. It's asking for trouble."

"Dad," Peter said, "that's illegal. There's no evidence that

AIDS—"

"In point of fact, *we don't know*," Roger said. "Peter, we're talking public health here. And until we can be *certain* how it's transmitted, society has every right to protect itself against these pederasts. AIDS is fatal. Let the deviates bugger each other all they want, but let's keep them away from healthy people. And don't tell me about these studies. I know who sponsors them. It's all the gay rights alliances and federations and whatever they call themselves. So, of course, the findings conveniently show that the gays are no threat to anyone. My ass."

"Bullshit," Peter said.

Roger reddened. "You're an expert on the subject, are you? How come you know so much about it? What's your data bank, your source, your authority?"

"Roger, Peter," Alicia cried. "Don't fight! You always go at each other like absolute *wolves*." She blew her nose, wiped her eyes, and handed Martin her glass. "Would you?"

"If I told you," Peter said, "you wouldn't believe me."

"And for good goddam reason. The way you waste your life . . . a man of your breeding . . . when I think of what you could have been—"

The argument had shifted ground.

Peter watched Roger. "You're ashamed of me."

Roger sat back. "I'm *not* ashamed. How could a man be ashamed of his own son?"

"You are, aren't you? A poor spirit in the gray twilight."

"Maybe someday when you have children of your own you'll understand. I wanted more of a life for you than you settled for." Roger stopped. "Sorry," he said to no one. "Didn't mean to blow up like that."

No one spoke or moved. Martin's stomach did flip-flops.

"Roger, you should be ashamed of *yourself*," Alicia said under her breath. "Peter barely out of a sick bed and you picking a fight with him." She swung her eyes to Peter. "Can't you two ever be civil?" She turned to Martin. "I'm afraid to have friends in when they're both there because they fight so, and I get mortified." She glanced from one to the other. "You'd think they'd outgrow it."

"Mom, please," Peter said. "I'm feeling kind of rocky."

"*Course* you are, darlin'," she said. She drained her glass and stood. "Hardly on your feet at all, then playing tennis and entertaining." She glared at Roger. "And *fighting*."

She started toward Peter, then stopped.

"Roger, honey . . ." She signaled him with her eyes. "Certainly good to meet you, Martin. I hope we can all get together again real soon." She pressed his hand. "Don't wait for Peter to bring you out. You come on out and see us. Peter, you get rested up and back on your feet. You don't seem at all yourself. I'd ask you to come on out home and stay but I know you wouldn't hear of it. If I don't hear from you by the weekend, I'll call, you hear?" She paused. "We'd better be on the road. So long, honey. You take care, now."

Roger mumbled something unintelligible, and they were gone. After the last sounds from the hall were swallowed in background noise, Martin turned.

Peter was still in the wing chair, his legs still crossed. He'd lowered his chin to his chest and closed his eyes. His face was misaligned, as if its two halves didn't quite fit together. A broken sculpture.

Martin undressed him, cleaned his face, neck, ears, and hands with cold cream and got him into a tub of hot water. While he soaked, Martin made the bed and washed the glasses.

"Ready to get out?" he called from the kitchen.

"Martin, would you come talk to me?"

Martin dried his hands and started toward the bathroom. He found Peter naked on the living room floor leaning his back against the bureau. The bottom left-hand drawer was open. Peter's head was bowed.

"You all right?" Martin said.

"Martin?"

"Yes?"

"Do you hate me?"

Martin knelt and put his hand on Peter's shoulder. "How can you ask me that?"

"Because I need to know."

"If I hated you, would I be here?"

"Do you forgive me for not telling my parents?"

"It's not my place to forgive you."

"Do you anyway?" Peter raised his head. He'd been weeping. "Martin, do you forgive me for being gay?"

Martin watched him.

"Do you forgive me for getting AIDS?" Peter's face contorted. "Do you think God forgives me?" Peter shook his head. Tears started down his cheeks. "I'm one of His mistakes."

Chapter 4

Cunniption's

Peter glittered with fever. Hundred and two. Martin telephoned Cohen. "What should I be watching for?"

"Nothing specific." Cohen paused. "Can't figure out what brought this on."

"He had a pretty emotional time with his parents last night."

Cohen grunted. "Okay, look, keep pumping liquids into him. Two aspirin every four hours. If he's not better by tonight, call and bring him in."

Peter turned down breakfast but drank orange juice. Martin set a glass, a pitcher of juice, and aspirin next to the bed.

"Drink this every time you can stand the thought of it," Martin ordered, "and take two more aspirin at about—" he checked his watch "—one or so. I put bananas and a sandwich in plastic wrap on the desk."

Peter growled and rolled over.

That evening, Martin found half the orange juice gone and the food untouched. Peter lay sleeping. Martin placed his hand on Peter's back. Damp. Peter stirred, opened his eyes.

"Hi," Peter said with unconvincing bounciness.

Martin felt his forehead. "How're you doing?"

Peter shrugged. Martin put on the perennial latex gloves, brought the thermometer, shook it, and put it under Peter's tongue.

"What time is it?" Peter slowly scanned as if the apartment were new to him.

"Don't talk. Keep the thermometer under your tongue."

"Tell me what time it is."

"Going on seven."

"I've really been catching me some Z's."

"Shut up, Peter." Martin withdrew the thermometer. "Down to a hundred point three."

"Broke this afternoon," Peter said. "Sweated an ocean. Maybe I could get you to change the bed and give me a bath before dinner."

"If you promise to eat a hearty meal."

"Promise."

"Who gets to define 'hearty'?" Martin smirked.

"I do."

"Nope. I do."

"All *right!* Anything for a clean bed. *Sacrebleu.*"

Martin put coffee on, drew Peter's bath, and donned fresh gloves. He helped Peter from the bed to the bathroom and stripped his damp pajamas from him.

"Get in," Martin said.

Peter watched himself in the mirror. "Everybody always said I was so sexy. They all said I had a big, beautiful cock." He looked down at himself. "You never said anything about it."

"Get in," Martin said.

"You think it's beautiful?"

"Stunning. Get in."

Peter sighed and climbed into the tub. Warm water slurped over his body. "You're making fun of me. And my cock."

"Peter, you're asking the wrong guy. Ask somebody who appreciates cocks."

"Nobody else to ask." Peter was still in the water, his eyes clouded.

"Can you wash yourself?"

"I'm feelin' mighty puny."

Martin lathered and began to scrub.

"I was right about my mom and dad, wasn't I?" Peter asked with a smug thrust of his chin. "They'd never forgive me, would they? My dad would hate me even more than he does now."

"He doesn't hate you."

"He's ashamed of me."

"I think he's disappointed, but I think he loves you."

Peter snorted. "What makes you think that?"

"The way he talked. And the way he watched you. I don't think a man can ever get over loving his child." He shrugged. "I bet your father's lonely."

"Dad?"

"Bet I'm right." Martin frowned as he lathered Peter's left arm. "You really did a job on your arm. Does it hurt?"

"What do you mean?"

"Your arm's all bruised. How'd you do it?"

"Where?"

"Here," Martin said, "on the outer arm." He traced the discolored spot with his fingers.

Peter grasped his arm with his other hand and turned the flesh toward him. He studied the bruise and squeezed it. "Martin, that's not a bruise. The color stays when you press on it."

"Then what—" Martin stopped.

"You think it's KS?"

Martin lifted Peter's arm and examined the splotch. Big as a silver dollar, purple and black.

Peter pulled his flesh toward him and looked again. "Jesus." His voice shook. "Let me get out. I'm cold."

Martin helped him from the tub.

"Will you make an appointment with Cohen right away?" Peter gaped at his arm in the mirror over the sink while Martin dried him. His muscles quivered. "And will you take that mirror down? And the one in the hall, too?"

Cohen made time for Peter in his schedule the following afternoon. He confirmed that the blotch was Kaposi's sarcoma.

They drove home from Cohen's office, up Connecticut Avenue, past Dupont Circle, up Rock Creek Parkway, through an ashen autumn rain. Colorless leaves swirled past the window. Peter sat in silence, then turned to Martin. "Remember when I asked you to take me to Cunniption's? Will you take me this week? Sunday afternoon, maybe?"

"You're too sick. You can't even exercise."

"I know, but I might not want to go later. After the KS . . . Or maybe I wouldn't have enough time left."

"Peter, you'll make yourself sicker."

"I know," Peter said.

Martin gritted his teeth and shook his head. "Okay. It's your life."

After lunch on Sunday, Peter dressed in his turtleneck, cardigan, and blue trousers. Martin insisted that Peter wear his overcoat, scarf, and gloves. Peter muttered under his breath about being treated like a child. They drove south on Connecticut through the wan sunshine to Dupont Circle and right on P Street.

"Park anywhere you can find a place," Peter said. "It's in the next block."

"How about if I drop you in front and go park?"

"*No!* You think I want to go in there by myself?"

After ten minutes of hunting, Martin finally parked three blocks from the bar. Peter called down curses on Martin's head for the extra weight of the overcoat.

At the entrance to Cunniption's, Martin helped Peter descend the three steps into the sunken, windowless barroom, lit by recessed pencil-beam spotlights in the ceiling. Between the long, straight bar on the right and a round piano bar on the left, Martin could barely make out a jumble of tables. Both bars were nearly full. Peter led Martin to a table for eight at the rear on the edge of the dance floor.

"Don't need one this big." Martin said.

Peter slipped off his coat and slid into a chair. "Never can tell."

Martin sat beside him. "Expecting somebody?"

Peter nodded with a closed-lip grin. "Called a couple of people and told them that I'd be here. That's all."

A waiter in suspenders and a straw hat arrived at the table. Martin ordered a draft beer. Peter asked for a glass of blush wine.

"You shouldn't be drinking," Martin said.

"I'll only wet my lips with it, to make it look like I'm part of the scene."

"Then order tonic water or something."

"I like the smell of blush wine."

Martin put his hand on Peter's forearm. "Don't do it, Peter."

"Get off my case."

Peter nodded to the waiter who returned at once with their drinks.

Peter got to his feet. "I'm going to the men's room."

Alone at the table, Martin reconnoitered. The men he saw were younger than he, stylishly dressed, and mostly good-looking. Nothing about them distinguished them as gay. On the other hand, he heard no female voices in the deep-pitched drone.

What if somebody made a pass at him? Would he know it was a pass? The men at the tables and the bars were laughing and talking, drinking and smoking, watching football on television—what guys always do at bars. Martin was surprised. He didn't know what he had expected. He hoped Peter wouldn't want to stay too long.

In the cramped men's room, a young man with green eyes and spiked hair the color of brightly polished copper primped at the mirror. Peter stood next to him at the urinal. As he finished, he snuck a look. The green eyes were watching him. Their owner smiled. His lips parted wide, showing off sparkling teeth. The corners of his mouth forced dimples into his cheeks and almost closed his eyes. The effect was *definitely* elfin. The face challenged Peter to mischief. That face. He knew that face.

"How can you see anything when you're smiling?" Peter said.

"So it is you. I wasn't sure." The man cocked his head. "Your name Peter?"

"Yes. And yours is—"

"Bruce. Didn't think you'd remember me."

"I remember you, but I can't remember where or when. Wait a minute. It was Christmas time."

"Between Christmas and New Year's."

"And we went to your place—up the street, right?"

"We read poetry. Paul Celan and Gerhardt Müller. And had fantastic sex."

"It was—what—two years ago?"

"Three. Really amazed you remember me." Bruce's eyes glinted. "I'll never forget you."

Peter felt his face redden. "Surprised you recognize me."

"You seem older. You've lost weight." Bruce frowned, his eyes now open and round, like a child's. "Are you sick?"

"Have been."

"Okay now?"

"I'm here, aren't I?"

"You with anybody?"

Peter did a double take. "You serious?"

"I thought that maybe we could get together if you didn't have a date or something. We could go to my place. If you're up to it. You . . . I don't know—"

"Then why're you propositioning me?"

Bruce's eyes glinted again. "I've got a good memory."

Peter pondered, shook his head. "First of all I *am* with somebody. Second, I'm not up to it. Actually, I'm quite sick. Third . . ." He put his hand on Bruce's arm. "I'm more flattered than I can tell you. I needed to have somebody think I was—"

"Sexy?" Bruce grasped his hand. The glint was gone. "What's the matter with you? I mean, what are you sick of?"

Peter hesitated. The time for hiding was past. He had to tell the truth. "AIDS."

Bruce didn't move. "My God."

"Hope I didn't shock you too much."

"No, no, not at all." Bruce shook his head and took a deep breath. "When were you diagnosed?"

"Over a year ago." Peter tried to think of something more to say. "Well . . ." He paused. "Good to see you again. You look great."

"Same here, so do you."

They left the men's room and headed away from one another, Bruce to the bar, Peter to his table.

"What took you so long?" Martin said.

Peter simpered. "Got propositioned."

Martin swallowed. "In the men's room?"

"By an old trick."

Martin scowled at the men's room door.

Peter smirked. "I didn't have sex in the men's room, you ninny. If you have to take a piss, go ahead. Nobody'll bother you."

"I'll wait."

Peter lit a cigarette. "Never been to a gay bar before? Don't worry. I'll protect you."

"Peter!" A man of Peter's age, slight and dark, dressed in overalls and a tee-shirt, an earring in one ear, bent toward Peter.

"Ron!" Peter said.

Ron threw his arms around Peter.

"Take a chair," Peter said. "Ron, this is Martin, my buddy from the Charbonne Clinic."

"Hi." They shook hands.

Ron sat, clapped his arm around Peter's shoulder, and jostled him. "So how *are* you?"

"Not so good, Ron. You look great." Peter raised an eyebrow. "You didn't tell Billy I was going to be here, did you?"

"You told me not to."

"Thanks. So what're *you* up to?"

Ron fairly bubbled. "Got a new job. Met somebody. He might be Mister Right."

Soon Peter and Ron were chattering like a pair of

chipmunks. They spoke confidentially, their faces close, their voices low. Martin had never seen this side of Peter. Catty, glib, gossipy. Swishy.

Peter lit a cigarette and signaled the waiter for another round of drinks.

"Peter, don't drink any more," Martin said close to Peter's ear.

"Don't bug me," Peter said.

Martin leaned back and frowned.

Two more young men arrived, repeated the joyful hugging, and took chairs. They were introduced to Martin as Joey and Kirk. Joey was big and blond. His chambray shirt, open almost to the navel, displayed ample blond hair. He was Martin's height but heavier. His jeans were too tight. Kirk was tall and willowy, with long dark hair, black snake eyes, and a day's worth of stubble. All three of Peter's friends were frenetic in their exchanges and periodic outbursts of falsetto laughter. They spoke a dialect all their own, stabbed each other with their fingers, and cackled over remarks Martin didn't understand.

"So when I went for the interview," Ron said, "I put my school ring on my left hand and turned the stone under. I asked if the medical benefits included maternity." Laughter. "And the dumb breeders hired me."

"And the new man in your life?" Kirk said.

"Oh, honey." Ron took Kirk by the bicep. "Peaches and cream. Bread and honey. Muscles and hair. Not much bigger than me. Blond. Not brawny enough for you, Peter. Not your type. 'Cept when you're having PMS and feeling mean and horny and being a chicken hawk."

"You should have brought him today," Peter said.

Ron's eyes flicked. "He wanted to come. Wanted to meet

you. He's heard so much about you, but he had to work."

"What's he do?"

"Computers. For HUD."

"They have him working on Sunday?"

Ron's eyes darted to the left. "Something came up. They called him. Emergency. Computer crash. Have to have everything up and running by tomorrow morning."

"And Ron," Joey said with false pity, "has to be home early so he can have dinner ready for his hubby when he gets in all hot and sweaty from the war, right?"

"Fuck dinner. I'll just greet him at the door in my feather boa. And three-inch heels. And nothing else."

Screeching laughter.

Peter smiled. "Sounds like—"

"How's that for being the dom?" Kirk cried.

Martin narrowed his eyes. The exchanges was getting feverish, as if Peter's companions were competing, compelled to ramp up the gaiety. Peter watched and listened, his smile fading.

Joey told them about a new bar he'd found in Southeast—called Suds 'n Stuff where the go-go boys strip while dancing on the bar. Kirk asked how it compared to Folly's. Better, Ron said. He and his boyfriend had been there last night.

Peter wasn't talking. His face was lined.

"You all right?" Martin whispered.

"Fine."

The conversation continued headlong. Kirk, Joey, and Ron got into competitive bar-hopping anecdotes, a can-you-top-this contest. Something phony was going on. The three were too dithery, too jubilant. Martin's gut tightened.

More drinks arrived. Peter was flushed. He was frowning and slurring his words. He no longer joined in the laughter.

Ron, Joey, and Kirk partied on.

"*They* don't know what a good time is, my dear," Joey was saying. "*They* wouldn't know a rush if they met one running bare-ass naked down the street." Kirk guffawed. Peter ground his teeth.

"And *that*," Ron said unnaturally deep in his voice, "is why they call us gay, big boy."

"Gay?" Peter said, his voice raw, his face red.

"Gayer than thou, honey," Kirk said. He poked Peter in the stomach and made a face at Ron. Hoots of laughter.

Peter gulped his wine. "*Gay?* Holy Jesus . . ."

Still smiling, Kirk turned back to Peter with a questioning look.

Peter slammed his glass on the table. Wine sloshed. "We're not the gays," he said though his teeth. "We're the shit of the earth, biological errors, mutants, at the genetic end of the line, with no hopes, no dreams, no salvation. Big fucking mistakes. God, we can't even reproduce."

The laughter died.

Peter lifted his glass with two trembling hands and sipped. The others watched. "I'm sorry. I don't know why I said that." His arms twitched. The glass slipped from his fingers. Blush wine splattered across the table into Joey's lap. He leapt to his feet. Kirk grabbed a napkin and dabbed at Joey's pants.

Peter scooped the wine back toward him. It ran over the side of the table and down his legs. Martin mopped with napkins.

"I'm really sorry," Peter said in half a voice. "Joey, have those cleaned. I'll pay."

He moved the palms of his hands through the wine on the table with helpless determination. "I'm so sorry. I didn't mean it."

Ron and Kirk gawked at him.

Peter's face crinkled. Tears started down his cheek. Eyes turned toward their table. The noise in the bar subsided. "Please, go ahead," Peter said in a broken whisper, "please, don't let me ruin the party." He blew his nose and lit another cigarette. "I'm sorry." He covered his mouth and sobbed.

Joey put his hand on Peter's sleeve. "What is it?"

"Nothing." Peter pushed Joey's hand away. "I'm sick, and I get teary sometimes. Ignore it and go on. *Please.*"

"Peter," Martin said, "you want to leave?"

"No, I want to stay. It's just . . ." He cried harder and leaned on Martin. "I want a future, Martin. They all have a future."

Ron gaped, mouth open. Kirk sent unhappy glances around the room. Joey bent in his chair, intent on wiping wine from his crotch.

"Peter," Martin said, "let me take you home."

Peter nodded, his face buried in Martin's shoulder.

"I'm so sorry," he whispered. "I'm so sorry." Now he was weeping out of control.

Martin put bills on the table and got Peter to his feet. He helped Peter into his coat, scarf, and gloves. He put his arm around Peter and led him through the room. They moved slowly, weaving past the tables, and ignored the silent upturned faces of handsome young men staring with curiosity, disapproval, and revulsion.

The following morning, Peter barely spoke. Martin let him be. Peter had been hurt. He needed time to get himself together. He'd come around. Like Catherine. Catherine would come around, too. In time.

During Martin's afternoon office hours, Catherine's smiling face in the framed picture on his desk made his heart hurt. Her hazel eyes and dark hair seemed to move in his peripheral vision. When he turned his eyes to the face, it froze again, as if caught in the act. He hadn't heard from her for nearly two months. How long was he supposed to wait? He pushed aside the mid-term blue books and picked up the telephone. The Registrar's office at GW told him the University forbade giving out the telephone numbers of students. Martin could write to her care of the University. Martin pulled a sheet of paper from his desk and took his pen in hand.

> My Dearest Catherine,
>
> So long since we have seen each other. I think of you every day and wonder how you're doing. I'm muddling through. My courses are going well, and I'm doing volunteer work. Other than that, no news, really.
>
> I don't know your telephone number. Please call me. I very much want to see you.

Martin read what he had written. He wasn't satisfied with it, but he doubted he could do any better. He scrawled "Love, Dad" at the bottom of the page.

That night Peter was silent and withdrawn. Tuesday morning, he spoke in monosyllables. Martin decided to wait. Peter would get over it sooner or later. Maybe he would even learn something from the experience.

By Wednesday night, Martin was worried. In the middle of washing dishes, he stopped and looked up. Maybe Peter wouldn't get over it. Peter might not live through the winter. Somehow the thought was new. Martin had known when he volunteered to be a buddy that he'd be taking care of someone who was dying. It was all right for "someone" to die. It wasn't all right for Peter to die. He loved Peter.

It was true. *I love Peter.* The way he loved Catherine. How in the hell did that happen? He put down the dishrag and the cup and gazed unseeing at the backsplash.

"The dishes won't wash themselves, nummy."

Martin jumped. Peter was standing in the doorway.

"Got awful quiet in here." Peter said. "Thought maybe you were playing with yourself." He giggled. "But no. You think you're the Sorcerer's Apprentice. Like Mickey Mouse in the movie. You think hard enough and the dishes wash themselves, right?"

"Guess I was lost in thought," Martin said.

Peter pulled up a dining room chair. "What about?"

"You."

"What about me?"

"That I care about you more than I ever meant to."

Peter's grin faded. He lowered his eyes.

Martin washed a plate. "Decided to talk to me again?"

"Sorry. Thanks for putting up with it."

"Forget it."

Peter lit a cigarette. "You didn't like my friends at Cunniption's, did you?"

"Don't think they're worthy of you."

"Come on. Who do you think I am?"

"You're Peter, and you're special, and I like you."

"And they're not special and you don't like them?"

"It's hard to explain."

"I'm no different from them, you know."

"I see that part of you is no different."

Peter blew out smoke. "And you don't like the bitchy part."

"Guess I like the bitchy part, too."

"You're not making sense, Martin."

"Guess not. Forget it." Martin rinsed a glass and put it in the drainer. "Can I ask you a personal question? Did you ever have sex with any of those guys?"

"Them? Shit, no. If I want sex with a man, I want sex with a man, not a queen."

"Oh." Martin gave up trying to understand. He dumped the dishwater. "Bath time."

Bathed and in fresh pajamas, Peter sat up in bed and leaned against the headboard. Martin pulled up the desk chair.

"My mother called today," Peter said. "She invited us both for Thanksgiving. Said she wanted to give us an early invitation so we wouldn't have any excuse. Told her yes. At the last minute I'll call up and say I'm sick or something."

"Peter, she'll be furious."

Peter frowned as though he hadn't thought of that. "Guess she will."

"What *do* you want to do on Thanksgiving?"

"Have dinner here, I guess. Wish we could invite someone."

"How about your friends—Kirk, Joey, and—what was his name?"

Peter huffed. "Forget it. Don't want them here. Anyone you want to have over?"

Martin thought of Catherine. "No."

"Martin," Peter said, "I never thought to ask you. Guess I took it for granted." He folded his hands. "I know it's a lot to ask, but holidays are the hardest of all for me. And I get scared sometimes when you're not here. Will you please spend Thanksgiving with me?"

"I'd love to. Will you let me buy the food?"

Peter turned down the corners of his mouth and nodded.

"Speaking of buying food," Martin said, "have you thought about what you're going to do when your money runs out?"

Peter turned away.

"Isn't much left, Peter."

"And you've been helping, haven't you?"

Martin raised his hands in denial.

"Yes, you have," Peter said. "I've been keeping track. I know what groceries cost."

"You could earn a little money if you want."

Peter humphed. "Doing what? Christ, I can't even stay out of bed for more than an hour or two."

"How about doing translations for me? I need good English renditions of *Das Lied von der Erde* and Strauss's *Four Last Songs*."

"Why don't you do them yourself?"

"I'm no poet, Peter."

"You can't afford my fee."

"Lincoln College can. I'll see if I can get you a contract. If that works out, I know a guy who's been wanting to get articles by Leichtentrit on musical forms into English."

Peter rubbed his lips together. "Thank you."

"Meanwhile, I bet your parents would help if they knew you needed money."

"I don't want them to know until after I'm dead."

"None of my business, but have you considered how that's going to make them feel?"

"Shit, Martin, you think they care? The worst problem they'll have is keeping the cause of death a secret."

Martin winced.

"They're as devoted to me," Peter said, "as my—what shall I call them?—toadies. The ones we met at the bar, you know? The same ones who don't call and don't come around, now that they know what I've got. They're scared shitless of me. Too frightened to say no when I called them and told them I'd be there. Too scared to give me a chance to speak, terrified I'd talk about dying or being sick. Could you see it?"

"I could see something. Wasn't sure what it was."

"That's why they behaved like harpies."

"If you thought so little of them, why did you hang around with them?"

"They were my entourage, them and a guy named Billy. They practically worshiped me. And I loved it. Used them for all they were worth." Peter huffed. "Pretty slimy, wasn't I? Using people right and left, trading on my looks." He frowned out the window. "I've been thinking about that the last couple of days. Figured nobody could ever love me because I was such a turd, so I screwed everybody out of everything I could get, to pay them back. I'm really a loser."

"Peter, no—"

"You don't know me. When you really get to know me, you'll see."

"That's hogwash."

Peter colored.

"You really believe," Martin said with a smile, "that after all I've been through with you I don't know you?"

"You only see the good side," Peter said with a toss of his head.

"Does that mean I'm into self-delusion or I lack perception?"

"You don't know the worst. I've used people. Even destroyed them. And I don't care at all. If I told you . . ." He stopped. "And recently, the last few months, I've really been into a self-pity thing. I'm sorry."

"Don't be."

"I want you to understand. I couldn't accept the idea that I was dying. I could feel my body withering. All I ever had was my looks. Never had any brains to amount to anything. No talent or trade."

"What about dancing?"

"I wasn't any good," Peter said. "I wanted to be, more than anything. I dreamed of the day I'd be a star. I'd dance at the Kennedy Center. I'd sneer at my small-minded father stuck in his functional office in Baltimore while I toured the world. Then I'd be ashamed of *him*." He shook his head. "No, it was more than that." He waved his hand back and forth as though erasing what he'd said. "I wanted to make a difference. I wanted to be at least a good dancer, because it was worth doing. I hoped maybe I'd even be a great one. Sometimes . . ." He leaned back and gazed into space. "Sometimes I think I really understand. I did have the talent to be a good dancer."

He turned back to Martin.

"I'm not bragging anymore, Martin. I mean it. Stella Adler said it right: 'It's not enough to have talent. You have to have a talent for your talent.' What I didn't have was the—I don't know—the guts, the devotion, the selflessness, the courage, the vision—all the things you have to have to be really good at anything. I wasn't man enough to be good."

"Because you're gay?"

"That has nothing to do with manhood. My father doesn't know that, but I do. He's right about me, anyway. I'm a no-account because I was never man enough to do anything worthwhile. He *should* be ashamed of me. I'm ashamed of myself."

Peter leaned against the headboard. Martin waited.

"Martin, there's still time left in this body. Precious time. There's still time for me to become a man. And I'm going to do it."

"How?"

"Don't know yet. Maybe helping others. I'd really like to help people with AIDS."

"Want me to ask the clinic if there's some kind of volunteer work you could do?"

Peter nodded. "I've decided to quit smoking, by the way."

Martin's mouth opened in surprise.

"So tonight," Peter said, "when you leave, would you take all the cigarettes and matches with you? And clean out all the ashtrays?"

"You're serious."

"Have to do it if I want to stay alive a little longer."

They sat looking at each other.

"How much longer do you think I've got?" Peter said.

"No idea. What does Cohen say?"

"He doesn't."

"You press him?"

"No."

"Maybe if you really insisted—"

Peter sighed. "He doesn't know. I'm the only one who knows."

Martin waited. "And?"

"Not too much longer."

"A year?"

Peter shook his head.

"Six months?"

Peter thought, then shook his head again.

"Three months?"

"Probably. If I take care of myself. Maybe even a little longer."

"How do you know?"

Peter studied his folded hands. "Every fall I always get to feeling full of piss and vinegar, always want to rush off and begin projects and stuff. This year, it didn't happen. I'm getting weaker. I can feel the rhythm of death in my body. I want to slow it down. I want to do all I can to lengthen the time I've got and to make the most of it. I want to be a man. I want to be able to look back, right before I die, and say, 'Nice goin', Peter. You done good.'"

He sighed and leaned back, as though he'd finished important work. "Tired." He closed his eyes. "Just to be able to say, 'Nice goin', son. You done good.'"

Part II

Beyond Reward

Chapter 5

The Johnny Connection

Seek not to reward goodness,
For goodness is beyond reward.

Peter repeated the lines aloud. Hàn Hsīng. He remembered
them from his book of Chinese writings. He'd sent the book—
anonymously—to Johnny Logan. Maybe it had given Johnny
pleasure. Maybe.

Peter propped himself on pillows and, through his window,
contemplated the scraps of lawn along Porter Street, dusted with
early November frost. He was frantic for a cigarette. *No.*

What did Peter know of goodness? He'd never even made it
up from vice to the neutral level. If he had, he'd have pretended
to be straight. He'd have married and had children by now. He'd
have a tedious little job, a little house in Fairfax, a little car.
And decency. The boring dignity of decency. Having it meant
nothing. Lacking it meant everything.

He ran his fingers along the bristles of hair at the top of his
head. Shorter than he'd ever worn it. Turned out Mort Gray was
a hair stylist. Mort minced a lot. Not Peter's type. No question
Mort was gay. Yet he touched Peter with the same respect Martin
did. Peter thought gay men didn't know how to touch that way.
Certainly he didn't.

He watched the frost disappear as the sun rose in the sky.

The only way he knew how to relate to other men was with his cock. Women, he touched with indifference. All except Sally, but she was a special case. No, he wouldn't think about Sally—

The phone rang. Peter started. He controlled his breathing and answered.

"Peter, this is Bruce Dushinsky. I ran into you last month at Cunniption's."

"How did you get my number? Oh, the telephone book."

"Never knew your last name."

"Didn't know yours, either."

They both laughed.

"No, actually," Bruce said, "Kirk gave me your number."

That son-of-a-bitch. I told him never to give my number to anyone.

"So how are you, Peter?"

"Not too bad. Some KS and trench mouth and something wrong with the left side of my stomach. Got lesions on my face. I can feel them. Mainly, though, I'm too weak to do anything. On a thousand medicines. They make me sicker than the diseases. And I quit smoking."

"Sounds rough. I'm sorry."

"Thanks for caring," Peter said, oddly touched.

"Least I can do."

No, it's not. You could have not called, like all the rest.

"You doing okay financially, Peter?"

"For now. Doing a little translation work for Lincoln College. On Medicaid. Charbonne Clinic helps out. So does my buddy, Martin, damn his hide. I'm getting by."

"Sounds like you're not depressed."

"Sometimes the days are so much alike I sort of lose track. I wanted to do volunteer work. Offered at the clinic, but they turned me down. Poetic justice. In my eleventh hour I turn altruistic and find out it's too late."

"I really called . . ." Bruce began.

Here it comes. Now we'll find out what he wants from me.

"I called because I want to apologize. When I found out you had AIDS, I ran away. I like you a lot, Peter, and I didn't want to make you feel any worse."

"Thank you."

"We should all stick together and not go running off. You probably don't understand. I got tested in August. Positive."

Peter chose his words carefully. "You probably won't get it. There's only a 5-to-20 percent chance."

"That's what they say now, but the probability numbers keep going up." Silence, then, "Peter, could I come see you?"

"Haven't had any visitors for a long time."

"Please."

"I have KS now, Bruce. It's a disfiguring disease."

"How bad?"

"I don't know. Martin took down all the mirrors."

"I don't care, Peter. I want to see you."

"No one's seen me since the KS started."

Bruce said nothing.

"I don't know," Peter said. "Let me think about it."

"My number is 333-9538."

After he hung up, Peter held the telephone in his lap. He turned his eyes to Porter Street. The frost was gone. Bruce wanted to help him. Bruce was so frightened about AIDS. Maybe Peter could help Bruce.

What was the reward for helping Bruce? None. Peter wasn't even up to the neutral level—where he could expect a reward— let alone up to the goodness level. *Goodness?* "Goodness is beyond reward." Peter wanted to laugh out loud. Goodness. *Nice goin', son. You done good.*

❖ ❖ ❖

As November progressed, the lesions spread. Peter traced them with his fingertips, wondered with a shiver what his face looked like. He watched the rose and orange leaves on the maples and locusts lose their color. The rain soaked them. The wind tore them. They dropped to the ground and joined the muck of the earth.

Every day, he sat in bed with the phone in his lap and witnessed the trees turning to skeletons. Every day, he thought about Bruce, but he didn't call him. He thought about Ron, Kirk, and Joey sometimes, and about Eric.

He thought about Billy, too.

One gloomy Wednesday morning, Peter dialed Billy's number.

"Hello?"

"Billy, this is Peter." Silence. "I called to tell you I'm sorry for hitting you." Billy said nothing. "Did I hurt you too bad?"

"Nothin' that didn't heal. It wasn't that. I thought you was my friend, that's all. The night you hit me was a long time ago, Peter. I forgot it already. You forget it, too, okay?"

Peter swallowed.

"I thought about calling you," Billy said, "but figured you wouldn't talk to me. You still mad at me for telling that hunk you had AIDS?"

Peter closed his eyes and lowered his head. "No."

"You have AIDS, don't you?"

"I lied to you and everybody else."

"How're you doin'?"

"Got KS now, Billy."

"Jesus. What can I do?"

Peter pursed his lips. "One thing, maybe. I wanted to ask about someone. Johnny."

"Johnny the piano guy? Peter, hate to tell you this, but he died—what?—seven months ago?"

"Kirk told me."

"Thought you never knew Johnny."

"Met him once." How much could Peter bring himself to tell Billy? "Did he have any family or a lover or anything?"

"Just his mom. He lived with her."

"What was her name?"

"Probably the same as his. Logan."

"Where did they live?"

"Virginia someplace. Alexandria, I think. What do you want to know for?"

"Maybe I'll call. Tell her how sorry I am."

"Peter, he died last March. Kind of late for sympathy."

"I just thought . . ." Peter gnawed his lip. "So how're you doing, Billy?"

"I got it, too, Peter."

Peter locked his throat.

"Only with me," Billy said, "it's not KS or pneumocystis. Toxoplasmosis. You know about toxo? It's, like, a brain disease—a brain parasite, they call it. Sometimes my doctors call it an infestation. They talk about things like 'new colonies forming.'"

Peter wished he had never called. "How serious?"

"Not going to get any better."

"Billy . . ." Peter began.

"Peter, cut it out. We're in the same boat. I'll be luckier than you, though. No pain or anything. 'Cept for headaches. I'll kind of lose control and fade out."

"How long?"

"Don't know. Not a year. Not too soon, neither. I'm still working. Can't remember things sometimes. Have trouble with numbers. Having some what they call coordination problems. They say that's normal."

Peter was silent, his eyes closed. "Can I help?"

"You already done it," Billy said. "You called me."

After the call, Peter shook his head. Billy diagnosed. Toxoplasmosis. Peter shivered. Far worse than anything Peter had ever heard of. Billy was pretty calm. No talk about boosting himself over the edge, no mention of three seconds or not being able to boogie. Billy, of all people, turned out to be strong in the face of death.

Martin wrote to Catherine once a week. No answer. No calls. Maybe he should leave her alone. She'd come back. In due time. *What if she doesn't? I've got to get her back.* One morning, before he left for Peter's apartment, he called Vivien.

"How are you, Vivien?"

"Busy. Negotiating on the construction of a new shopping center near Paris."

"Sounds like you're doing fine."

"Yes." Her voice let him know that she didn't have time to talk.

"I called to ask about Catherine. How's she's doing?"

"She told me you two weren't speaking," Vivien said, her tone almost clinical.

"*She's* not speaking." Martin took a deep breath. "How is

she?"

"Settled into GW. Excited about her classes. Of course, she never talks to me, so most of what I'm telling you is surmise."

"Why didn't she accept the MIT scholarship?"

"She never actually refused it. The offer is still open. She mentions it sometimes, but I discourage her. I don't think she should be that far from home. I'm her sole support, in case you've forgotten. Actually haven't seen her for a couple of weeks. She came home one weekend middle of last month to get her stereo."

"You haven't tried to call her?"

"I've been terribly busy myself. Trying to sell the house, in addition to everything else. It's really too large. Need something more compact."

Martin's chest hurt. The house in Potomac. The home he and Catherine had worked so hard on.

"Trying to get ready for the trip abroad," she said, "and close a deal in Louisville at the same time. And Catherine doesn't like me to call her, especially at the library. I wouldn't give her as much spending money as she thought she ought to have, so she got herself a job at the Gelman Library on campus."

"How does she have time?"

"She only works from six to ten Monday and Wednesday nights."

"I've written to her," Martin said. "She hasn't answered. Thought I might telephone her."

"Do whatever you think best. She's angry with you. Frankly, Martin, I think she's never forgiven you for breaking up the marriage."

"I didn't break up the marriage."

"We could spend the morning debating the point," Vivien

said, "but I'm due at the office. In any case, it's perfectly *clear* that *Catherine* sees you as responsible for the destruction of our marriage because of Hedda. If you were going to sow your wild oats, Martin, you might have done it in a way that didn't hurt Catherine so."

Martin clenched his teeth. "Vivien, will you give me Catherine's phone number?"

He could hear her breathing. Finally, she said. "I'm not sure she'd want me to."

"Please, Vivien. I want to talk to her. Please."

Another silence, then, "Very well. She's in room 408, Morton Hall. Call the hall number and dial 408 after the message."

"Thank you."

"Good luck. You may tell her I gave you her number. Anything else?"

"No."

"It's always good to talk to you, Martin," she said. "Please call any time."

She probably wasn't being sarcastic. It was her surface graciousness, her patina of detached kindness, without roots or depth. It went with the general air of competence. He hated her for it.

That afternoon at the office, Martin found the number for Morton Hall and called.

"You have reached Morton Residence Hall on the campus of The George Washington University in Washington, D.C. If you know the number of the room you wish to contact, enter it now. Otherwise, stay on the line and an operator will assist you."

Martin dialed 408. The number rang. A young female voice answered.

"This is Catherine's father. May I speak to her?"

Long pause. "Let me see if she's here."

The sound of a hand over the mouthpiece, indistinct voices. Then, "She's not here right now."

"Ask her to call her father?"

After he hung up, he waited. Hours passed. No call. The next day, Martin tried again. Same result. He tried every day. Catherine was never there.

Saturday, Martin arrived at Peter's apartment early.

"Today," he announced, all grins, "we're gonna make this place *shine*. In the Navy, I learned all about the aesthetic, practical, and moral beauty of hot soapy water. Today I'm going to demonstrate. In the bathroom and kitchen."

Peter turned on his side. "What brought all this on?"

"Haven't given the place a thorough cleaning in the three months I've been coming here. Doesn't smell good. Needs sterilizing. Besides, I'm full of energy."

"Your problem is not enough sex." Peter extended his arm and examined his fingernails under raised eyebrows. "*Tu es trop hôrné.*"

"Wouldn't be surprised but what you're right," Martin called from the kitchen. "Just once I'd like to have enough sex and see what it's like."

"Might take all the starch out of you. As it were."

"As it were. Still like to try it."

Peter giggled to himself. He felt a rush of affection for Martin.

Martin came from the kitchen drying his hands. "Forgot to tell you. I showed your translations to a professor in German lit.

She liked them. Wants to know if you've ever done any of Paul Celan's poetry. She's going to call you."

Peter moistened his lips and rubbed them together. "Martin, how do I look? Am I gruesome?"

Martin shrugged.

"Pretend you don't know me," Peter said. "How bad do I look?"

"Very sick."

"Ugly? Horrifying?"

"You'd scare people who are already scared."

"I've got death written all over me, don't I?"

"It's not that bad, Peter."

"Does the KS make me into a character from a horror movie? Do I make you sick?"

"You don't make me sick."

"Martin, *tell me*. Is the KS horrible?"

Martin looked away. "The KS is horrible, yes."

"I like you," Peter said with a grim smile. "You've got the balls to tell me the truth."

"Peter, how you look doesn't matter to people who care about you."

"But people who knew me . . ." Peter rolled his head. "If they back off in horror . . . I don't know if I could take it." He bit his index finger. "Maybe I'll try an experiment. I could invite somebody over, a guy named Bruce. He propositioned me in the men's room at Cunniption's."

"A guy after you for sex isn't going to react well to seeing you sick."

"He's hot for my bod, all right. Or at least he was. Mainly, he likes me, you know? He's the only person who cares about me."

"What about your parents? What about me?"

"You're different. You *have* to like me. You're my caretaker. And my parents *have* to care about me. Bruce likes me, that's all. Or at least he said so."

"He told you that in the men's room when he was propositioning you?"

Peter laughed. "No, he called a while back. Could we invite him for dinner—next Saturday?"

"Suits me."

While Martin was scrubbing the kitchen floor, Peter telephoned Bruce. Bruce accepted the invitation. "And, Peter," he said. "Thank you for trusting me."

Peter slept while Martin scoured the bathroom. After lunch, Martin pulled on latex gloves, gave Peter a back rub, dressed him in fresh pajamas, changed the bed, and put him back into it.

"Can we talk for a few minutes?" Martin said.

"If I don't fall asleep. So comfortable, thanks to you."

Martin drew a deep breath. "You have to think about some things soon. For example, have you thought about a will?"

"I don't have anything to leave anybody."

"Your furniture, the television, your clothes, personal items—you know, like letters or photos. If you don't have a will, your parents will presumably get your stuff."

"Can't afford a lawyer."

"The clinic will pay. And how about a living will?"

Peter grunted with revulsion.

"Know what they are?" Martin asked.

"Sort of. Instructions for taking you off machines when—"

"Not exactly. It's a legal document telling doctors what measures to take to keep you alive."

"Like what?"

"Respirators, catheters."

"God," Peter whispered.

"If you don't have a living will, your doctor and your parents will decide."

Peter turned on his side and put his face into the pillow. "No way do I want my mother and father deciding."

Martin said nothing. Peter looked at him. "There's more?"

"Toward the end, I won't be able to take care of you alone. The Hospice of Saint Anthony can admit you, but you have to agree to palliative care."

Peter's stomach froze. "I can't think about that."

"And you have to decide what kind of a memorial service or funeral you want."

"Dear God. I'll think it all through. Right now, I want to sleep for a while. I'm worn out."

Martin rose. "Sleep fast, 'cause I need to vacuum."

"You callous bastard!" Peter hissed. "Don't you care at all? You go through a conversation like that and throw it off like it was nothing?"

Martin colored. "I never meant—"

"Next time think of what you mean before you say something like that!" Peter rolled on his other side, his face away from Martin. "God."

"Wait a minute," he heard Martin say. "You're accusing me of being callous?"

"Leave me *alone!*" Peter said.

"Peter, you're way off track."

Martin was breathing heavily. After a moment Peter heard him gather the dirty sheets, pick up the basket, and leave for the laundry room.

Left alone, Peter permitted himself to weep aloud.

◈ ◈ ◈

When Martin came back from the basement, Peter was asleep. Martin folded the clean clothes at the dining room table. He knew from his buddy training that a buddy has no business passing judgment. A buddy never loses his temper. A buddy's emotions are his own business, not to be unloaded on the patient. And yet . . . When he was giving Peter his back rub, he'd found three more lesions.

The balled socks rolled from his hand. Upset? The problem went deeper than that. He'd lost Catherine. Now he was going to lose Peter. He felt the familiar hurt grip his stomach and move up into his chest.

A light knocking at the door startled him. When he opened it, he saw a young woman in a green wool coat and black boots. Her hair was long, straight, and blond; her eyes hazel; her cheeks pink from the cold.

"Is Peter Christopher in?" she said.

"He's ill. Can I help you?"

Her eyes grew large and round, her mouth turned down at the corners. "Is he too sick to have visitors? Are you a doctor?"

"A friend. He's asleep, that's all."

"Martin?" Peter called.

Martin chuckled. "He's awake now."

She followed him in. Peter, still tousled with sleep, sat up.

"Sal?" he said in an unfocussed voice.

"Are you mad that I came?"

"No, Sal, Sal—"

He reached to her. She knelt by the bed. They clasped each other with murmurs and sniffles.

"Sal, Sal, Sal." Peter clung to her, eyes closed, and rocked from side to side. She leaned back. They surveyed one another.

He took her hands in his. "You're so beautiful."

She handed him a tissue. "Blow your nose."

"You blow yours, nummy." They blew together. Peter glanced at Martin and laughed. "Martin must wonder what the fuck's going on. Sal, this is my best, truest, most loved friend, Martin."

The girl, still on her knees, turned toward Martin.

"Martin," Peter continued, "this is Sally Murdoch. Sally and I go way back. Haven't seen her for—what?—six, eight months, Sal?"

"Not since last March."

"You look *great*." His smile faded. "I don't look so good, do I?" She shrugged. He pointed to the lesion now covering half his nose. "I was afraid you wouldn't recognize me. Would you like a cup of coffee or anything? Martin, would you be an angel and make coffee?"

"Of course." Martin was trying valiantly to be an angel, but he was feeling put upon. He pushed the desk chair toward Sally. "May I take your coat?"

He hung her coat in the closet and went into the kitchen. He was not, after all, Peter's servant. Why was it that as soon as Peter's old friends showed up, Martin was expected to be seen and not heard? Peter and Sally chattered and giggled. Martin felt a rush of shame. He should be sharing Peter's happiness. Instead he went on smarting.

"So where are you working now?" Peter was asking her.

"Still at Walter Reed. It's no better. You know the military."

Martin returned to the living room. He pulled up a chair from the dining room table and sat at the foot of the bed.

"Still living in Laurel?" Peter asked.

"Sharing a condominium in Potomac. Moved in April."

"Seeing anyone?"

"Just dating around."

They watched one another.

"Did you test positive?" Peter asked.

She shook her head.

"You said you'd call me," Peter said. "I called your number. They said you'd moved. Walter Reed wouldn't put calls through to you."

"I didn't want to talk to you, Pete. I was upset." She gave him an apologetic wince. "How are you?"

"I have my ups and my downs, but the downs win in the long run. Right now, I'm having a good period. Actually gained a little weight."

"If nobody minds," Martin said, "I'll go on with my work while we talk."

"Go right ahead," Peter said without looking at him.

Martin moved back to the dining room table, finished folding the clean clothes, and put them away. He watched Sally. Her hair shimmered when she moved her head. Her skin glowed with health. Her eyes twinkled. She moved her body with efficiency—like a dancer. No. Like a nurse. She was so supple, so fresh, with the unconscious grace of youth, like . . . Of course. Like Catherine.

Peter and Sally drank their way through a full pot of coffee as they talked through the afternoon. Martin left them long enough to make a shopping run. When the groceries were put away, Martin asked Sally, "Will you be staying for dinner?"

"Would you, Sal?" Peter said.

"Don't want to tire you."

"If I get tired, I'll send you home."

Sally insisted on helping. She told Peter to rest and joined

Martin in the kitchen. While Martin started on the rice and vegetables, she washed the flounder and greased the broiler pan.

"Have you known Peter long?" she asked.

"Since August. Guess you know his physical status."

"That he has AIDS? Yes."

"That's why I'm here. I'm a volunteer with the Charbonne Clinic."

She stopped. "You're his buddy?"

Martin nodded.

"I thought . . ." She trickled lemon juice and olive oil over the flounder. " . . . that you and Peter were, um, lovers."

"I'm not gay."

She looked up. "You're not? Oh."

She lifted the pan with one hand, bent at the waist like a gymnast stretching, and slid it under broiler in the oven. Martin had to admit she had a lovely young body. Awfully pretty in that position.

"I never met a straight buddy before," she said as she raised her torso back to a standing position. She leaned back her head and gave it a quick shake. Her hair rolled away from her face like a departing wave. "Bet you hear a lot of tales. Does Peter have to explain what things mean?"

Martin shrugged.

"Yeah," she said, "you're a buddy, all right. Bound to silence like a confessor. Do buddies have to take a vow or sign up to a code of conduct, like, you know, the Hippocratic oath or something?"

Martin chuckled. "No."

Over dinner, Peter and Sally took turns telling anecdotes. Sally had shared this apartment with Peter. And they were obviously close. Yet Peter had never mentioned her.

After ice cream and coffee, Martin dabbed at his mouth and put his napkin on the table. Trying not to sound fatherly, he said, "Time to get Peter into his bath and ready for bed."

"Can I help?" Sally asked.

"Let her help," Peter said. "Sally's a nurse, Martin. She took care of me for a while."

Sally nodded. "I can give Peter his bath while you finish your coffee."

"Fine," Martin answered, embarrassed at his possessiveness. "Or better, I could get the dishes out of the way and change the bed."

She stood. "Super."

"Actually, he's plenty strong enough to bathe himself."

"No, I'm not," Peter said. "Sal will have to bathe me." He looked from one to the other with a smile intended to beguile angels.

"Whatever you say, Pete," she said as if singing. "I'll go get the bath ready, then show you the way."

"Latex gloves on the toilet tank," Martin said.

"Got it." She disappeared into the bathroom. They heard water running.

"If I didn't know better," Martin said, "I'd say you were on the make for that young lady."

"Really?" Peter said, immensely pleased.

Martin washed dishes to the accompaniment of laughter from the bathroom. He gave himself a stern talking to about unjustified and demeaning jealousy. He had just finished the bed when Peter shuffled into the room in clean pajamas, leaning on Sally. She walked beside him, her arm around his waist. In the middle of the room, he sagged, steadied himself, took a deep breath, and made his way to the bed. As Sally stripped off her gloves, he settled himself on his pillows and gave her a look of pure love.

"Can't tell you how good it's been to see you," he said. He reached for her hand. "Come and see me again?"

"As long as I'm welcome, Pete."

"Always welcome, Sal." They hugged. "Martin, will you drive Sal home?"

Sally turned to him. "I hate to ask, but I don't live near a metro stop, and it's so late for the bus."

Martin and Sally said good night to Peter, let themselves out, and headed downstairs. In the elevator, she was silent. When they reached his car, she took tissues from her purse.

"You okay?" Martin said.

She nodded and blew her nose.

"Where are we going?" he said.

"Sorry. Potomac. North on Connecticut. I'll tell you when to turn."

"Where did you and Peter meet?"

"He waited on a banquet for the National Association of Nurses at the Shoreham a year ago last May. As soon as I saw him, it was all over. He reminded me of Michelangelo's *David*."

"He must have been quite handsome when he was healthy."

"You don't know the half of it. I called and asked him out. I'd never done that before."

Martin shot a look at her.

"It never dawned on me he was gay," she said, "until one night in a bar he walked off and left me for a pair of tight jeans—male variety."

"Rough way to end a relationship."

She shook her head. "I was so much in love I couldn't stop. In July, I moved in with him." She paused long enough to blow her nose again. "First I found the calendars with male nudes. Then the cock rings and posing straps and dildos and pictures of Peter naked in the crudest positions. A couple of times a week he'd stay out all night. I was frantic. Once he left on Friday night and didn't come back until Tuesday. We fought. His defense was that I knew what he was when I asked to move in. Martin, I didn't know. I never met anybody so self-centered."

Sally gazed into the night, as if lost in thought. Martin drove in silence.

"Once in a while," she said from her reverie, "he'd do something beautiful. For his dad's birthday, Peter bought him the most gorgeous set of silk ties you've ever seen. He couldn't afford them. And when somebody he knew was diagnosed with AIDS, Peter sent him a book of Chinese poetry—a book Peter had paid a fortune for and really cherished. I persuaded myself that underneath the prima donna was a man who could learn to love if somebody gave him a chance. By that time he was already getting sick."

She peered ahead.

"He'd been having night sweats and occasional fevers all summer. I didn't know it until I moved in, but he was having a hell of a time with diarrhea, too. The thrush started. Three days later, his fever was up to a hundred and four, and he could barely breathe. I called an ambulance. He was in GW hospital three weeks. They diagnosed him with pneumocystis—and AIDS. When he came home, I took care of him, and he got better and went back to work. And it started all over again."

"You weren't infected?"

"I had no way of knowing until last spring when the test came out. Peter called me and insisted that I take it. He made the arrangements and paid for it. I tested negative."

"Thank God."

"We hadn't made love since he started really feeling sick, toward the end of August. I stayed with him through the winter, despite everything. Our relationship was strictly platonic. We weren't even sleeping in the same bed. I'd given up all my dreams of settling down with him, getting married, having kids. In March of this year, he had his second bout of pneumocystis. He almost died. That's when I left."

She turned toward Martin.

"I stayed with Peter when I knew he was gay. I stayed after I'd given up all hopes of marrying him. I stayed even when he treated me like trash. I couldn't stay and watch him die."

Following her directions, Martin drove into a cul-de-sac lined with town houses. "Sally, are you going to hang around and watch him die after all?"

"If he wants me to."

"Why?"

She looked down with an embarrassed laugh. "I've gotten over my addiction. When I was in love with him, I wanted to possess him, to own him, to *have* him all for myself. After he broke my heart, I grew up. Now he's more like a sick child than the man I once loved. Now I can help him."

"Guess Sal told you about us last night," Peter said over breakfast Sunday morning.

"Didn't leave much out."

"Martin, did you ever try to make love to a woman and you couldn't get it up?"

"Never been my problem."

"I couldn't get it up with Sally. She had to help a lot. I didn't even know I could do it with a woman. I kept thinking, 'Boy, if Dad could see me now.'"

"Your parents ever meet Sally?"

"I bragged about her. Sort of wish my dad had known we were sleeping together."

"Why didn't you tell him?"

"He would have thought it was funny if I told him I was proud because I fucked a woman." He sipped his orange juice. "I love Sally."

Martin stopped eating.

"Not the way she wanted," Peter said. "Not like a man loves a woman. I love her for what she is. I didn't know until last night. She'd never believe it. Do you believe it?"

"Yes."

Peter pushed his plate away. "What did she tell you?"

"That you were lovers. I don't know why everybody tells me everything."

"That's because you're from the clinic. Everybody kind of sees you as a professional, cool and detached. They know you're trained not to blab."

"How come you know so much about it?"

"I've had friends die of AIDS. I knew their buddies."

Martin took a bite of toast. "Is it harder for you—having watched others die?"

"Guess it made me more scared. Not of death. Just of dying." He sat immobile and frowned into the distance. "Martin, I apologize for acting like a queen yesterday."

"Me, too. I'm so used to being around you and kidding and everything. Sometimes I kind of forget how sick you are."

"You plan to stick around, when I, you know—"

Martin nodded.

"Aren't you scared?"

Martin nodded again.

"Sometimes I'm afraid you'll get disgusted and leave," Peter said. "Will you stay with me while I die? So I don't have to be alone? I'm so scared."

Martin put his hand over Peter's. "I'll be here."

Peter wiped his eye with his index finger. "I wanted you to drive Sally home so that she'd tell you about her and me. I didn't know if you'd be back this morning. I put her through hell to see if she'd stay with me. To *prove* that she really loved me. And if she did love me, that would prove how worthless she was, and I wouldn't want her." He blew his nose. "I figured I had AIDS before I was diagnosed. We had sex after that. I risked her life. Didn't care at all." He stopped, looked at Martin. "I wanted you to know, so if you're going to be shocked and leave, you can do it now."

Martin swallowed hard.

Peter took a deep breath. "I need to go to bed. I'm very tired."

He stood. Martin helped him back to bed, got him settled, then cleared the table and drew water to wash the dishes.

"Martin?"

Martin left the dishes, went to the living room, pulled up the desk chair, and sat by the bed.

Peter's eyes were fixed on the ceiling. "I *have* to tell you something. If you're going to leave, I want you to leave now." For a moment he said nothing, then he whispered, "I killed someone. I had sex with him after I got out of the hospital last fall. He got AIDS and died."

"My God."

"And I didn't give a flying fuck. He was only twenty-two.

And very sexy. He didn't know anything about how to do it.
Had to show him. Taught him a lot. I gave Johnny AIDS."

"Johnny—"

"His name was Johnny Logan."

Martin closed his eyes and turned his face away.

"I never saw him or his family or anything," Peter said. "I
never did anything to help. I never let on that I knew him. I
told you I wanted to visit the mother of a man who died. It's his
mother. If I can find her. Maybe if I talked to her . . . You think
there's any way she'd forgive me?"

Martin stood. He was trembling.

"Martin?" Peter said.

Martin walked to the bathroom. He flipped the tap and
rinsed his face with cold water.

"Martin?" Peter said again.

Johnny Logan.

Martin heard a thud. He got control of his breathing and
walked back to the living room. Peter had gotten out of bed and
fallen. He lifted himself on his elbows and looked up.

"I knew Johnny Logan, Peter," Martin said. Peter's face froze.
"He was my student, the one I told you about."

Peter lowered his face to the floor.

"I need to go home, Peter."

Peter raised his head. "You coming back?" His sunken blue
eyes were open so wide that the irises were ringed by white.
"Please come back."

He touched Martin's shoe. Martin pulled his foot away. Peter
put his face to the floor.

"Get up," Martin said. "I'll help you."

"You're not going to leave?"

Martin helped him to his feet.

"You're going to stay?" Peter said.

Peter sat on the bed and put his arms around Martin's neck. Martin slid him into the bed and pulled the covers over him.

Martin returned to the kitchen and finished the dishes. He needed to vacuum. He needed to finish cleaning the bathroom. He needed to think.

Chapter 6

Lasagne

Martin came back to the apartment on Monday morning. He cooked Peter's breakfast. He said little. Peter didn't speak. By nine, Martin was ready to leave for the campus.

Through the day, as he taught, held office hours, and corrected assignments, Johnny's face stalked him. In the halls, the classrooms, the offices, he saw Peter prone on the floor, his eyes large, the pupils blue moons in a sky of white.

That afternoon, Martin telephoned Mort.

"You said if I ever needed anything I could call you," Martin said. "I'm going to ask them to take me off the case, Mort. I'm sinking."

"Why didn't you say something at the meeting? Have you talked to a counselor at the clinic?"

"Shit, no, don't have time."

"Big, grown-up man. You can handle yourself without any help, right?"

Martin said nothing.

"How about if we get together for a couple of beers?" Mort said. "Tonight, after my guy's asleep. Meet me at The Lexicon on H Street, up from the White House. Nine okay?"

That night, Martin parked on 17th Street near Lafayette Square. He had never been in The Lexicon before. The interior was lined with bookshelves and furnished with heavy oak tables, each lit by its own brass lamp with a green shade. The bar was half filled with men drinking draft beer. No women.

"This a gay bar?" Martin asked Mort when they were settled at a small table in the corner.

"Sure. Wrinkle bar."

Martin blanked.

"You know, a watering hole where the older crowd gathers," Mort said. "Thought you knew the place."

"Never been here before."

"How could you have missed it?"

Martin took a deep breath. "I'm not gay, Mort."

Mort sipped his beer. "Why—if you don't mind my asking—"

"Long story. You were right. It's getting harder. Last night Peter told me he had sex with a guy—a kid really. Gave him AIDS. The kid died."

"God almighty."

"I knew the kid, Mort. You went to his funeral. Johnny Logan. Peter killed him."

Mort studied his mug. "So now what?"

Martin wanted to weep. "They should get Peter another buddy. I can't stand to be with him. I can't stand to see him getting sicker, day after day. Today I tried to be kind to him, but I kept seeing Johnny's battered face." He laughed. "I thought Johnny had been in a fight. I didn't know about KS back then."

"Would Peter care if they assigned somebody else?"

"I don't know. He depends on me. He asked me to be with him when he dies."

"He must love you."

Martin reared.

"Couldn't you hang in there," Mort said, "for Peter's good?"

"I don't know."

"If you stick with him, you'll have to forgive him."

"Who am I to forgive him?" Martin said.

"We're all forgivers."

"I don't think I have it in me to forgive him. You didn't know Johnny."

"You can't take care of someone you're holding a grudge against. You'll end up torturing him." Mort took a slug of his beer. "Martin, your job is not to judge Peter. Your job is to help him die. That takes a lot of love."

Martin turned his face away and closed his eyes.

"What would Johnny have wanted?" Mort asked.

Martin saw Johnny's ruined face. "I don't know. The last time I saw him, he was raging." He wiped his nose. "I don't know what to do. I can't bring myself to quit, and I can't stand to stay. I'll think it all through again." He let his shoulders droop. "At least I got to talk about it. You're good at this. How did *you* get into this kind of work?"

Mort shrugged. "My lover contracted AIDS, and I found out I couldn't ignore the epidemic any longer. He died three years ago. You're lucky. Most of us buddies are looking in the mirror."

"Who're you taking care of now?"

"Kid named Billy. Peter knows him. They had a falling out a while back." Mort's face turned weary. "Billy has toxoplasmosis. Probably won't live much longer. He doesn't realize how quickly his mind is failing. Sometimes for a few hours, he becomes lucid and he sees what's happening. Talks about killing himself. That's when it really hurts."

"Billy's not your first patient?"

"My sixth. I helped with others."

"God. I don't see how you do it."

"I'm in for the duration," Mort said.

"What happens after Billy?"

"They want me to be a team leader." Mort hesitated. "Want to be on my team?"

"Sure."

"Have you thought about what it's going to be like after Peter dies?"

Martin lifted his mug to his lips and let beer roll over his tongue and down his throat.

"Won't be fun," Mort said. "Sounds to me like he's become pretty important to you."

Martin watched the random motion of patrons at the bar. Someone was laughing. Set high in the wall, a flickering television commercial hustled the new Pontiac Fiero.

"Don't mean to dwell on it," said Mort. "Just—you ought to be prepared."

Martin let his body sag. "I get the message."

"Martin, will you call me if you need to talk?"

"Yes. Will you call me? I'm a good listener, too."

Mort's face turned bittersweet. "I'm gay, Martin."

"We can still talk like human beings."

"Deal," Mort said.

From The Lexicon, Martin walked across Lafayette Square, past the White House, up Pennsylvania, to the GW campus. He'd put off confronting Catherine long enough. Since it was Monday night and not yet ten, he'd do it now. While he still had the reinforced backbone the talk with Mort had given him. Catherine would be working at the library. At ten, she'd go back to Morton Hall. He'd wait for her there.

As he walked down 21st Street, he passed students wrapped

in coats and mufflers and gloves, their breath steaming in the cold air. When he caught a glimpse of faces in the light of the street lamp, he wondered at their youth. They ought to be home with their mothers, not living on campus in the middle of Washington. Three boys stood on the sidewalk in front of the concrete steps to Morton Hall, arms full of books and workout bags and tennis shoes. "Don't take it if Harrington's teaching it," one said. "Four papers in the first four weeks."

Martin glanced at his watch. Just ten. He climbed the steps to the double glass doors. A security guard was at a desk in the lobby reading a paperback. If Catherine spotted Martin, she might bolt. He went half way back down the steps and into the shadow of the trees beside the entrance and waited. The three young men didn't notice him. The wind was rising. He pulled his coat tighter around him.

A girl in an oversized charcoal coat and red scarf with a Walkman plug in her ear hurried down the street and turned in. As she started up the steps, Martin recognized her walk.

"Catherine—"

She snapped her head toward him.

"It's Dad," he said.

"What do you want?"

The conversation among the three men stopped.

"I want to talk to you."

She stumbled backwards. "No."

Martin dashed down three steps and took her arm. "You didn't return my calls."

She pulled her arm free. "Leave me alone."

"Give me five minutes."

"No."

Martin felt a hand on his arm. One of the boys was on the

steps beside him. "Hey, man . . . " he said.

"I'm her father," Martin said.

"Make him leave me alone," Catherine said.

The kid tightened his grasp. "Beat it, old man."

The glass doors swung open. The security guard came onto the steps. "What's the trouble?"

"She's my daughter," Martin said.

"Leave me alone!" Catherine said.

"Sir," the security guard said, "you heard the lady."

"I only want to talk to her," Martin said. The young man yanked his arm. Martin stumbled down a step. "Take your hands off me."

Catherine darted in. The security guard followed and closed the doors behind him. The lock clicked. The young man let go.

Three more people, two students and an old woman, had stopped on the sidewalk.

"I'm her father," Martin said in a shaking voice.

No one answered. Martin straightened his coat, tried to sneer at the upturned faces, and walked down the stairs past the young men. He turned up 21st Street and hurried toward Lafayette Square.

Peter awoke. Rain came down in waves. He listened. No sounds in the apartment. Martin hadn't come back from his classes yet. Tuesday. Martin wouldn't be back until six. Peter reached for the telephone. Could he make himself do it? He had to. He dialed Billy's number.

"Billy?"

"This is Mort. Friend of Billy's."

"Mort Gray? This is Peter Christopher. Is Billy there?"

Vague sounds in the background.

"Hullo?"

"Billy?"

"Hello, Pe . . . uh, Peter."

It was Billy's voice, but the speech was odd.

"Did I wake you?"

Long pause.

"I wasn't a . . . uh . . . asleep."

Something was wrong. "Are you okay, Billy?"

"Not as g-good as I, uh, was, Peter. I've had, like, setbacks, you know?"

"Jesus, Billy," Peter said.

"I can't, uh, talk very good, so I'll put Mort on."

Before Peter could protest, Billy was talking in the background. All Peter could get was "old friend, so it's, uh, okay."

"Hi, Peter. I'm Billy's buddy. Small world."

"Small fucking world. Mort, is Billy okay?"

"He's having severe problems now, Peter. It's the toxo. Sometimes he has trouble talking."

"Is he bedridden or anything?"

"Mostly. He's having a good spell right now."

"Mort, how long does Billy have?"

Mort's voice was flat. "Probably not until Christmas."

Peter shivered. "Does he know?"

"Yes."

"Tell him I love him."

Mort spoke away from the receiver. Billy said something.

"He says he's always loved you, Peter," Mort said.

❖ ❖ ❖

Peter sat on the examining table and waited. Cohen was writing in Peter's chart. Cohen was so sexy. Masculine to the core without being macho. Tall, angular, and good-looking in a Latin way, with a winning smile, flashing dark eyes, and a light frosting of silver at the temples.

But Peter dreaded The Look. In it were grief, despair, frustration, and defeat. It always went with words like, "that's all we know how to do," or "medical science hasn't solved that problem yet." When The Look took over, Cohen's eyes got large and round, deep and dark. His face lost its animation. His mouth became solemn, even sorrowful. When Peter saw The Look, he knew Cohen was going to tell him something he didn't want to hear.

Cohen put down the chart. "The x-ray doesn't show much. We could test further, but it doesn't really matter. If it *is* KS lesions in the stomach lining and the intestines, we could go to radiation or chemotherapy. Both are pretty rough. I'd rather not get you involved in either one unless things get worse. Now, about the canker in your mouth, it's KS. I'll give you something for it." He paused. "You're not acting like your normal feisty self. What's up?"

Peter set his jaw. "How long have I got?"

Cohen squirmed with his hands. "Awfully hard to make a forecast with a disease like this."

"A year?"

Cohen hesitated. "Do *you* think you've got a year?"

Peter shook his head. "Six months?"

"Don't know. You could hit a plateau. Hard to say."

"I really kind of need to know."

"Patients sometimes take my statements as a prediction and die at the appointed time. I want you to live as long as possible."

"Three months?"

Cohen slumped. "Probably. Maybe more, maybe less. Depends on so many things."

Peter sighed. "Thanks."

The Look again. "Sorry I couldn't help more."

On the way home, as they waited in the traffic at Dupont Circle, Peter turned to Martin. "I want you to go in with me the next time I see Cohen. I've decided to make a will. I want to name you as my executor and give you power of attorney if I'm incapacitated. And I want to set up a living will. Don't want a funeral. I want to be cremated, then a memorial service with you and a couple of others. I'm going to sign a notarized letter saying all that."

Martin kept his eyes on the road, his face immobile.

"The reason for the letter," Peter went on in a quavering voice, "is to protect you. Because I want to ask you to promise me that *you'll* see to it that what I ask gets done. My parents will be like cornered cheetahs."

Martin nodded.

Peter stared straight ahead. "I know what I'm asking. I'd rather lay this on someone else. You really going to stick around, Martin?"

"I don't know."

"You've changed. It's Johnny, isn't it?"

Martin said nothing.

Peter nodded. "We do pay for our sins, don't we?"

"Give me time."

"I don't have much time. How grim. How ruthlessly grim. Turns out life's fair after all."

That night, Peter ran a fever. He didn't call Martin. The fever stayed with him through the following days. At night it went up.

Peter's stomachache became constant. He couldn't force himself to eat. His breathing was congested. By Saturday, he was so weak that Martin had to help him to the bathroom.

"How about if I call Bruce and tell him not to come tonight?" Martin said over Peter's uneaten lunch.

"Don't," Peter whispered. "Might be the last chance I'll have to see him."

Bruce arrived shortly past seven. He went to Peter's bedside before he took off his coat. "Hi."

Peter smiled up at him and watched for signs of shock or revulsion. Instead, he got the Bruce grin, all dimples and crinkles.

"I'm still sure you can't see anything when you're smiling," Peter said. "Did you meet Martin?"

"We introduced ourselves," Martin said.

"Take off your coat," Peter said. "Martin, help me sit up."

"I brought you something." Bruce put a round pink cake-saver in Peter's lap.

Peter lifted the lid. "You made it?"

Bruce nodded. "German chocolate."

"My favorite." Peter gave Bruce a doubtful look. "How did you know I liked German chocolate?"

"You told me," Bruce said. "Don't you remember? It *was* three years ago. Do you remember that I told you I like to cook?" Peter shook his head and frowned. Bruce smiled. "Never mind."

"You look great," Peter said. "I had good taste, didn't I?"

"Not as good as mine," Bruce said with his elfin grin.

"I don't look as good as I used to." Peter waited for a reaction. No sign in Bruce's face.

"Are you hurting?" Bruce asked.

"I have stomach problems now, but I hadn't been hurting much before. Feeling lousy most of the time. How about you? No symptoms?"

"Nothing at all."

Martin silently squirmed as the dinner conversation languished between Bruce's anecdotes. No one talked while they ate. Peter nibbled to be polite. He accepted a piece of German chocolate cake but didn't eat it. After coffee, which Peter couldn't drink, Bruce said he should be going. He knelt by the bed and put his arms around Peter and squeezed him.

"Let me show you the way." Martin went to the door with Bruce.

In the hall, Bruce stopped. "My God, I had no idea. He's gone downhill so fast. His face . . . Anything I can do?"

"Come and see him sometimes," Martin said. "He was so pleased."

Bruce nodded. "God. I can't get over it. He was so beautiful before he got sick. When he walked into one of the bars, the conversation in the room sort of dried up and blew away while everybody ogled him. And he was wonderful in bed. Or maybe you already know."

"No," Martin said, forcing back his irritation, "I never—that is, I'm not gay."

Bruce stepped back. "I'll . . . stop by."

"Probably only for short visits—say half an hour."

"Right."

❖ ❖ ❖

The day after Bruce's visit, Martin spotted a new lesion above Peter's cheekbone. It pushed his left eye out of place.

His face more and more resembled an out-of-focus Halloween skull mask randomly daubed in black and purple, its oval shape stretched and flattened. Hideous was too kind a word for it. And the bones in his torso protruded against skin spattered with lesions. Swallowing hurt—now even the mildest food caused sharp pain in the stomach. The next Tuesday, Martin waited next to Peter while Cohen scrutinized x-rays against the translucent pane of white light on the wall. Two new internal lesions. One in the stomach and one in the right lung.

"It's time to start radiation," Cohen said. "I can refer you to a fine radiologist with plenty of experience in KS. His office is in this building. I'll ask him to give you priority. This shouldn't wait."

"Jesus," Peter said.

"It has to be done, Peter."

"They pump you full of beams that kill your cells, right? Burn them to death."

"Only the cancerous ones. Normal cells have more resistance."

Peter shook his head. "No."

Martin tensed.

"I know it's not pleasant," Cohen said, "but it's the best way."

"No."

"Peter, you'll shorten your life."

"No machines," Peter said. "Isn't there some other way?"

"Not with your stomach in such bad shape. Chemotherapy is out."

Peter shook his head.

"It's up to you, of course," Cohen said. "I'd strongly advise—"

"No machines."

Cohen opened his mouth and drew in breath to speak. Then he hesitated. He closed his mouth. His face sagged. His eyes darkened. His mouth was solemn. "It's your life and your decision. If you stick with your choice, I can help with the pain."

Peter sat rigid in the VW on the way home. Too much bad news all at once. When they pulled up in front of the pink portico of Quebec Towers, he shifted his body to confront Martin. "I want to invite Sally and Bruce for Thanksgiving. And a guy named Billy. I have to know if you're still going to be here. I can't do it by myself."

Martin, his gloved hands still on the steering wheel, surveyed the dirty windshield.

"I want you to know that I don't blame you," Peter said. "What I did was unforgivable. I didn't expect you to come back Monday morning. Each day I wait for you to tell me that your replacement is on his way."

"I don't know what I'm going to do," Martin said in a monotone. "I'll tell you when I know."

Peter peered at the parking lot. "Thank you. I didn't think you were holding out on me. You're too decent for that. Can you stand being with me until after Thanksgiving? Holidays frighten me. I don't want to be alone. I'm too sick to go to somebody's place, but I can't invite anybody unless you fix dinner. I couldn't ask a new buddy to take that on."

"I couldn't get a replacement before the beginning of the month. I'll be here."

Peter didn't move. "Thank you. Nothing I could do would be enough to repay you. A scumbag like me never deserved a buddy like you."

Martin opened the car door. "Let's get you in and park the car. While you're in your bath, I'll fix something to eat. Then I have to go to campus."

That night, before his third bath of the day, Peter called Bruce and Sally and asked them to Thanksgiving dinner. Both accepted. Peter called to see if Billy might be well enough to make it. After he hung up, he held the phone in his lap. "Mort says Billy's too sick," he told Martin. "Billy's gotten to the point that most of the time he can't speak at all. Can't even walk."

Wednesday morning of the week before Thanksgiving, Martin awoke in a sweat. He'd been dreaming he was making love to a sleek brunette with green eyes and the smell of Scotch between her breasts. Then Peter was crying for help. Peter kept pleading, weeping. Martin turned away from him, but the woman was gone.

On his way to Peter's, Martin stopped at the Peoples Drug on Connecticut to buy Maalox.

"We're out of it," the blonde behind the prescription counter said. "Why don't you try Bromo-Seltzer?"

Martin ground his teeth. "The patient has stomach lesions. He needs Maalox."

"Pepto-Bismol works just as well." The phone on the counter rang. "'Scuse me." She picked up the receiver and snatched a pen and order pad. "Uh-huh. Uh-huh. If the tab on the vial says 'no refills,' we'll have to contact the doctor. You have his number?"

Martin tensed his jaw muscles. The woman behind him in line sighed. The man behind her coughed.

"In that case," the blonde said into the phone, "you'd better talk to the pharmacist. Can you hold?" She pushed several buttons on the telephone and hung up. "It's Mrs. Clancy, Leon," she called over the partition and rolled her eyes. She turned back to Martin with a toss of her head. "Now, you wanted—"

"Maalox."

"We're out of it."

"You told me."

"How about Milk of Magnesia?"

"The man's dying," Martin said with acid softness. "He wants Maalox."

"Tell him they're all the same anyways."

"Goddammit," Martin shouted, "the man's dying. If he wants Maalox, you give him Maalox." He started out of the store.

"Jeez," the blonde said, "you'd think *I* killed him or something."

Martin crouched in the car, his teeth clenched. He was sweating. He needed to back off.

When he arrived at the apartment, his stomach knotted, he found Peter sitting up in bed, his mottled face washed, his hair slicked back.

"Good morning, bunkie," Peter said.

"Morning. You're better."

Peter shrugged. "Now you see it, now you don't."

"Can your stomach stand coffee?"

"*Sans autre.* What do you think I am, an invalid or something? What's for breakfast?"

"Whatever you'd like."

Peter examined his nails at the end of his extended arm. "Lasagne. *C'est très chic.* I have a recipe. In the desk, top drawer." He looked expectantly at Martin. Martin went to the desk and raked through paper clips, rubber bands, dead ballpoint pens, pencil stubs, and ragged papers until he found a tattered card, pock-marked with ancient flecks of tomato sauce.

"That's it," Peter said.

"'Lasagne' is misspelled. You spelled it ending with an 'a.' The word is plural in Italian. If you spell it with an 'a' on the end, it means a single piece of pasta."

"For Christ's sake, Martin. This is no time for an Italian lesson."

"It's wrong, goddammit."

Martin sat in the desk chair and read through the recipe. He was a buddy. What the patient wanted took precedence. His own feelings were irrelevant. The recipe seemed easy enough. He checked his watch. No morning classes. He had enough time. "Can you wait while I go to the Safeway?"

"I beg you," Peter said, gracious to the fingertips, "take as much time as you need. As you may have ascertained, I am a gentleman of leisure."

At the Safeway, Martin bought ground beef, pasta, ricotta and Parmesan cheese, French bread, and garlic. And Maalox. Back at the apartment, he replenished Peter's coffee and set to work. Following the instructions he preheated the oven and prepared the meat sauce and cheeses and spread them on the pasta in layers. He put his creation in to bake. When he returned to the living room, Peter was sound asleep.

For forty minutes, Martin read the *Lincoln Log*, the school newspaper, at the dining room table. Peter's translation of Gerhardt Müller's experimental poetry was printed side by side with the German text. Martin flinched at the poetry, but the translation was surprisingly good. Half way through a long poem about a shoe's ruminations on his owner's libido, Martin checked his watch. He put the paper on top the refrigerator and took the lasagne from the oven. It smelled rich, tangy, and mellow all at once. He spread garlic butter on the sliced French bread and put it under the broiler. While it toasted, he cut out two servings of lasagne. Finally he retrieved the bread, burning his fingers and swearing under his breath, put the whole works on a tray and went to the living room. "Lasagne's ready."

Peter opened his eyes.

"Sit up," Martin said. "What would you like to drink?"

Peter growled, rolled over, and faced away from Martin. "God, it smells ghastly."

"Come on. I spent two hours fixing this. So sit up and eat it."

"The thought of it makes me nauseous."

"Peter, wake up. You're dreaming or something. This is the lasagne you asked me to fix."

Peter rolled onto his back. "Sorry. I really can't eat that."

"What are you talking about?" Martin said, his voice rigid.

"The smell makes me want to puke."

Martin's voice softened to a rasp. "Let me get this straight. You had me go out and buy stuff to fix you a special breakfast. You snooze while I'm cooking. And now you're going to turn up your fucking nose at it?"

Peter's voice broke. "Will you please leave me alone?"

"Goddammit!" Trembling, Martin picked up the tray and carried it to the kitchen.

"Martin? I'm sorry."

Martin was too angry to stop. He scraped the lasagne out of the baking pan into the garbage pail beneath the sink and crammed the garlic bread in on top of it. Still shaking, he slammed the pan into the sink and whipped the hot water on full force. Water splattered the wall, the floor, and Martin himself before he could turn the tap off.

"Martin? What are you doing?"

"Throwing it out," Martin yelled.

Peter began to sob. Martin stood by the sink, his eyes closed. Finally, he took a dish towel from the rack and walked to the living room, drying his hands as he went.

"Martin, I'm sorry. I can't eat right now."

"So what am I supposed to do? Say 'oh, that's okay'? Chalk it up to experience? You think my time counts for nothing? You think I can come in here and cook for a couple of hours any time you get a craving for something and smile happily when you don't eat it?"

Peter tried to slide himself into a sitting position but failed. Martin made no move to help him.

"Please forgive me," Peter said through his sobs.

Martin raised his head and breathed through his open mouth. "You think that your being sick is an excuse? We're all going to die, you know. Not just you. You're not all that special."

Peter coughed between sobs and gasped for breath. Unable to speak, he looked at Martin, his eyes resigned. His eyeballs disappeared upward inside his eyelids.

"*Peter!*" Martin sprang to the bed, pulled Peter to him, and thumped his back. Peter's coughing and sobbing subsided. He lay limp in Martin's arms, an oversized, bony rag doll. Martin laid him on his back, pulled the covers over him, and sat in the chair by the bed. Peter's breathing became quiet and even.

Martin phoned the college to cancel his office hours. A little after two in the afternoon, Peter opened his eyes. He mouthed Martin's name.

"I'm here, bunkie," Martin said. He put his hand on Peter's forehead.

"Martin," Peter said in a hoarse whisper. "I didn't used to care what I did to people. Didn't care at all. That was when I was so bad I'd lost myself. I'm not that bad anymore. I've learned from you. Now it's too late. I can never be forgiven. Johnny . . ."

Martin, blinking back tears, sat on the bed and pulled Peter into his arms. "I know it's not much. I'm not God or anything. But I forgive you."

Chapter 7

Something to Live For

When Lincoln College closed for Thanksgiving, Martin spent his waking hours at Peter's. He and Peter treated each other warily, as if each were still bruised, the skin still tender to the touch. Neither mentioned Johnny. Yet Johnny was there in the apartment with them, like an unseen burglar.

Martin was so engrossed in Peter's pain that he barely felt his own. He saw with a kind of grainy clarity that there was no turning back. So he searched for an opiate. He found it in hard physical labor. He scrubbed and waxed and laundered and cleaned until no surface was dull, no fabric soiled. He set aside the day before Thanksgiving for final cleaning and meal preparations. He got to the apartment early so he could vacuum and dust and sweep and wash away the streaks he'd missed in the window by Peter's bed. Following Fanny Farmer's directions, he baked a pumpkin pie. He checked the turkey, bought on Monday, to make sure it would be completely thawed by the following morning. After lunch, he drove to Pearson's on Wisconsin Avenue for champagne and two bottles of Nuits-Saint-Georges. On his way back, he picked up potatoes, onions, butter, flour, and cream.

After dinner, Martin bathed Peter and helped him back to his bed. As Martin stripped off his gloves and smoothed the covers, Peter gave Martin a pleading look. "I have a *big* favor to ask."

"Shoot."

"I want to see someone. While there's still time."

"Who? I'll call and—"

"She wouldn't ever come here."

"Then how—"

"I want to go and see her."

"Peter, you're in no shape to be out visiting."

"I have to do it."

"Who is it?"

"Johnny's mother."

Martin stood straight.

"Will you help me?" Peter said.

"Let's ask Cohen if he thinks you should be out and about."

Peter shook his head. "You know what he'll say."

"Let me call her. See if she'll come here."

"She won't."

"Let me ask her."

"No."

Martin sighed. "Peter, I couldn't in good conscience let you do it. You're too sick."

"What I do is my business, not yours. Besides, you took me to Cunniption's."

"That was a big mistake. And you weren't so sick then. Tell you what. If Cohen says it's okay, we'll do it."

Peter rolled on his side, his back to Martin.

"I'm sorry, Peter."

Martin went back to the kitchen and drew dishwater. He hated to disappoint Peter, but what could he do? Seeking the balance between what would help Peter live a little longer and letting Peter do what he wanted was like caring for a toddler who knows no fear.

When the counters were swabbed and the floor mopped, Martin dried his hands and went to Peter's bed.

Peter flopped onto his back. "Are we still friends?"

Martin drooped with relief. "Sure. You need anything? Juice? Coffee?"

"No. I didn't want to start Thanksgiving with you and me mad. I get so scared sometimes. Will you hug me?"

Martin enfolded Peter in his arms, as he had Catherine when she was little. Not much left of Peter. And what there was shivered in Martin's arms. He arranged Peter's body in the bed and plumped the pillows. "You want me to spend the night?"

"You're not my type," Peter said.

"I don't like leaving you alone."

Peter attempted a tired grin. "Get out of here. I want some peace and quiet. How can I rest with you around, you noisy bastard? Always vacuuming or clanging pans or slamming the front door when you take the garbage down."

"I'll put the phone by the bed from now on. Call me if you need anything."

By the time Martin got back to his own place in Wheaton, it was nearly nine. He was stripping off his shirt when the phone rang.

"Martin?" Vivien sounded like she was in a tunnel. "Martin, I've been trying to reach you all day."

"Where are you?"

"Paris. The negotiations are dragging on. Doubt we'll be finished before the weekend."

Martin pursed his lips. "Thanksgiving in Paris. Not as good as April, but—"

"Spare me your failed attempts at humor."

"That's nothing. You should see the really noble things I've failed at."

"Martin, this is a transatlantic call."

"And I'm screwing it up."

"Screwing up . . . speaking of things you've failed at."

"I can't take all the credit for that," Martin said. "The little woman was a big help. You know what they say, 'Behind every great man stands a woman telling him he's wrong.'"

"You *were* wrong."

Martin shook his head. Among Vivien's charms was her total inability to see humor. "So what's up?"

"I'll get straight to the point. I've been trying to reach Catherine since yesterday. She's expecting me to pick her up when she gets off work to take her home for the holiday."

"Jesus, Vivien," he said, then wished he hadn't.

"I don't have time to listen to criticism from you, of all people. The point is, can you have a cab pick her up at ten o'clock in front of Gelman Library on the GW campus?"

Martin checked his watch. "I guess so."

"Have the cab take her to the new house. Tell her to get a locksmith. She doesn't have a key."

"You've moved?"

"Just before the trip."

"You didn't send me your new address."

"Have your lawyer get with my lawyer—"

" . . . and we'll do lunch."

Vivien clicked her teeth. "Tell Catherine there was nothing I could do."

"No," Martin said. He groaned. Poor Catherine.

"What?"

"Nothing you could do," Martin repeated.

"Tell her I'll call her as soon as I get back," Vivien said.

Martin's grin turned to a full-blown smile as he hung up. *Cab my ass.* He raced to the shower, rinsed, threw on clothes, and was out the door.

◆ ◆ ◆

A piercing wind, cold and angry, whipped the rain and battered the VW as Martin drove into the District. He pulled up in front of the library early to be sure Catherine wouldn't have to wait in the downpour. Shortly after ten, she stepped through the glass doors, suitcase and purse in hand, and sloshed through the puddles across the sunken cobblestone courtyard and up the short flight of stairs to the sidewalk. She walked to the curb, sheltered her face with her hand, and peered down the street through the pelting drops. Martin left the car. She stepped back.

"Catherine," he shouted over the downpour. "It's me. Dad."

She looked into his face, her expression blank, her lips parted. She took another step back.

"Your mother couldn't make it," Martin said as he wiped the water from his eyes. "She's still in Paris."

She searched up and down the street again, as if expecting to see her mother.

"Come on," Martin said, "get in the car before we both drown."

"No."

"Catherine, for Christ's sake, get in the car!"

She glowered at him and glimpsed the locked door to the library. Finally, she put her suitcase in the back seat and got in.

Martin ran to the driver's side and slid behind the wheel. "She asked me to tell you there was nothing she could do."

She didn't move. "I can't go home. Can't get in. And the dorms are closed until Friday."

"Stay at my place. Or get a locksmith at ten o'clock the night before Thanksgiving in the pouring rain."

She dried her face and hair with a handkerchief. "Take me to a hotel."

"Come back to my place. I won't bother you."

"I'll stay in a hotel."

"You have any money?"

She opened her purse, sorted through objects he couldn't make out in the dark, and closed it again. "Twelve dollars."

"You have a credit card?"

"Mom won't let me." She clicked her teeth together through open lips. "Will you give me some money? I'll pay you back as soon as Mom gets home."

"I don't have enough."

She resumed clicking her teeth.

"Don't *do* that," he said louder than he meant to.

"What?"

"Click your teeth. I've been trying to break you of that for years."

"I only do it when I'm upset."

"It's bad for your teeth."

She didn't answer.

"You'll have to come back to my place," he repeated.

"I don't want to."

"You have no choice."

She glared at him, opened the car door, and started to get out.

"*Catherine!*" he yelled, "*get back in here and close the door.*"

She paused, startled.

"You can treat me like shit if you want to," he said, "but I won't allow you to wander the streets with no place to go."

She wavered.

"Get in!" he yelled.

She got back in the car, closed the door, and leaned her head against the window.

He watched her for a moment, started the car, and drove through the empty, shining streets.

They passed Washington Circle and descended to Rock Creek Parkway, now leafless and bleak. The creek, swollen from the rain, raged in the darkness. He glanced at her. She sat contemplating the road ahead of her.

"How have you been?" he asked.

She shook her head.

"Studies going okay?"

She nodded.

"Still seeing that boy you told me about?"

She shrugged.

By the time they pulled up in front of his house, the rain had subsided to mist. It clung to them as they left the car and walked to the porch. Before Martin unlocked the door, he heard rock music. Young male voices sang about a woman named Rio who dances on the sand.

The music was louder when Martin opened the door. Craig, unshaven, in shorts, a sweat shirt, and rubber clogs, lolled on the sofa. A lit cigarette smoked in an ashtray. An opened beer stood on the coffee table in front of him. A rumpled *Playboy* lay in his lap. When he saw Catherine, he put out the cigarette and sat up.

"Hi."

Martin put down Catherine's bag. "Craig, this is my daughter, Catherine."

Craig bustled to his feet, stepped to the stereo and lowered the volume, and turned to Catherine. He offered her his most engaging smile.

"Hello," he said, his voice unnaturally husky. "I've heard so much about you."

Catherine swept him with her eyes.

"She'll be staying for a couple of days," Martin said.

Craig smiled more broadly. "How about a beer or something? You both look like you went swimming with your clothes on."

"No, thanks," Catherine said.

"Let us get settled first," Martin said. He picked up Catherine's suitcase and headed through the hallway to his room. Catherine followed. He went in and flipped on the light.

"You can have the bed," he said. "I'll sleep on the sofa."

He rummaged through the top shelf of the closet. Under boxes of summer clothes, he found the spare pillow and blankets. "Have you eaten?"

"Not hungry."

"I'll fix you something." He headed for the door. "Why don't you take a hot shower? Bathroom's at the end of the hall."

Martin put on a fresh pot of coffee. He could hear the shower. He nodded. She wasn't as sure of herself as she pretended to be at all of eighteen.

He stood before the open refrigerator and scratched behind both ears. Two six-packs, a bottle of Taylor Rosé, mustard, tomatoes, meat wrapped in butcher paper, and leftovers—all belonging to Gary, Craig, and Stan. The mayonnaise was Martin's, and so was the bread and lettuce, bought last week. In the meat drawer he found a pound of bacon, also his. He went to the living room.

"Who do the tomatoes belong to?"

"They're mine. Help yourself." Craig scratched under one armpit. "Catherine's quite a girl. You didn't tell me."

"Hands off. She's very upset right now."

Catherine appeared in the kitchen while Martin was arranging cooked bacon on tomatoes. She wore a nubby bathrobe that had once been neon pink. Her hair hung in wet strings.

"BLT on toast," he said. "That's all I had the makings for."

She nodded.

"You want coffee?" he asked.

"Beer."

"Catherine, you're only eighteen."

"Eighteen is the legal drinking age in D.C."

Martin worked his lips. "All right. It's in the refrigerator."

He set her sandwich before her at the table and sat opposite her. She ate while he drank coffee.

Craig wandered in. "Don't let me disturb you." He put an empty can in the trash under the sink and took another beer from the refrigerator. "How long are you staying?"

"Until Friday," Catherine said without looking at him.

"Great." Craig waited. "No one else is here. Gary and Stan are gone until the weekend. Let me know if there's anything I can do."

Catherine ate in silence.

"Stereo too loud?" he asked.

"No," Martin said.

"Anything you'd like to hear? I've got the Michael Jackson album."

"No, that's okay," Catherine said.

"Well," Craig said, "enjoy your dinner."

He flashed his smile again and sauntered back to the living room.

"How's your mother these days?" Martin asked her.

"Fine."

"See her often?"

"No."

"Bet she misses you."

"I doubt it."

"Catherine, she does care about you, you know. You're her daughter."

"Big deal."

"*I* miss you."

She finished her sandwich.

He watched her. The skin beneath her eyes was blue. "You look tired. Are you all right?"

"I'm fine."

"Studying hard?"

She nodded.

"Grades good?"

"A's."

"All A's?"

She nodded.

"I'm impressed. I never got all A's."

She shrugged, wiped her mouth with her napkin, and took a swallow of beer.

He finished his coffee. "I really do miss you. Do you believe that?"

"I don't know."

He rose and poured himself coffee. "Can I get you anything else?"

She shook her head. "What are your plans for tomorrow?"

He took a chair. "I'm fixing Thanksgiving dinner for someone."

"Here?"

"No." He hesitated. "You'd be welcome."

She gave him a patronizing look. "Don't you think that would be a bit awkward? Dragging your grown daughter along would get in the way of screwing your lady friend. Your cocksmanship might be in jeopardy."

"*Stop it*," he said with a flash of anger. "Who the hell do you think you are?"

She reddened. Her eyes widened.

The music from the next room stopped abruptly. Craig ambled in, smile in place, beer in hand. "I'm heading downstairs to bed. Have a good evening."

He offered Catherine one last leer and walked past them to the basement door at the end of the kitchen. The door opened and closed, and clogs slapped down the steps.

Martin filled his lungs and let the air ooze out. "The person I'm having dinner with tomorrow isn't a woman. It's a man dying of AIDS. I'd like to be having dinner with a woman. I'd like to end the day in bed with her. I've done that before, and I'll do it again. I'm not a monk. You'll have to accept that, Catherine. Parents are people. We don't like to sleep alone."

"Mother doesn't mind."

"Her passion isn't men. It's not even people. That's why we're not married anymore."

Catherine reddened again. "That's *not* why. She threw you out because you were sleeping around."

"Wrong. The marriage was over long before that. Hedda was a result, not a cause. She wasn't the only one, by the way. She was the last one."

Catherine's eyes opened wide. "You bastard. How can you sit there and tell me that?"

"What have I got to lose?" Martin said with a shrug. "You might as well know all of it. Your mother didn't throw me out because I was unfaithful. She didn't care about that. It was the scandal. *That* she couldn't forgive."

Catherine got to her feet. She was trembling. She went to the sink and stood with her back to Martin.

"I still love Vivien, by the way," Martin said. "Not as much as I used to. I've gotten over hating her for the most part. Someday I won't care about her at all."

"God almighty," Catherine said without turning.

"We're just people, Catherine. Your mother and I each have vices we haven't been able to overcome. At least I'm learning that I've got them. Your mother still doesn't know that success is an addiction."

Catherine spun to face him. "If all that's true, why didn't you fight her during the divorce? Why did you cower like a beaten dog with your tail between your legs?"

"Because I *was* a beaten dog. You don't understand. Hell, I'm only beginning to understand myself. I loved your mother. When I saw that she had no time for me, I tried different things to shock her into realizing she might lose me. I underestimated her indifference to me and her devotion to her career. Finally the thing with Hedda did it."

"You want me to believe you calculated all that out," Catherine said, "while you were screwing other women?"

Martin shook his head. "If you'd asked me at the time, I couldn't have told you why. Now I think I understand. I know it was shabby, but it's true."

"Jesus Christ," she said. "And you have the gall to get mad at me? Who in the name of God do you think you are?"

"Your father, that's who!" he shouted, rising.

"And what about me?" she cried. "Growing up with these two *hideous* people who don't give a damn about me. I know she never cared about me. Don't you think I know that? But you, *you* . . ." Her eyes filled with tears. "I loved you. I trusted you." She sobbed, still furious. "You dropped me. Walked away. So you could be with your . . ." Her voice grated. " . . . *women.*"

"Catherine, no . . ." He stepped toward her.

"You never cared about me at all. *I hate you.*"

She wobbled, turned, and leaned on the side of the sink. Her voice rose, then shattered. "Why did you leave me? Why, why, why? Oh, Daddy . . ."

She tensed. The sobs stopped. She wiped her face with her hands and wavered, still shuddering, then groped toward a roll of paper towels on the counter. She tore one off, mopped her face. Back at the table, she sank into her chair and straightened her back. "Can I have another beer?"

"I'll have one, too."

He sat across from her, opened their beers, and scratched behind one ear.

Catherine clutched her beer. She wouldn't look at him.

"I'm sorry I yelled at you," he said. "About clicking your teeth, I mean."

Catherine's mouth showed the first hint of good humor he'd seen all night. She blew her nose. "We'd better go to bed."

Carrying her beer with her, she rose and headed to the bedroom. He followed.

"I'm going to the bathroom," she said as she opened her suitcase. He nodded.

When she returned, he'd changed to pajamas, something he

never wore, and donned his bathrobe.

"I'll set my travel alarm for five," he said at the door. "Have to get going early because I have a complete Thanksgiving dinner to fix. What are you going to do tomorrow?"

"Hang around here, I guess."

"I wish you'd come with me."

"I don't feel like acting the part of your devoted daughter. Who's going to be here?"

"Craig, I guess."

"Just him and me?"

He could hear her brain figuring.

"Could you . . ." she began. "Could you stay here tomorrow?"

"Wish to God I could. I promised Peter I'd fix dinner. He's dying, Catherine."

"Couldn't someone else do it?"

"He doesn't have anyone else."

"Why are you doing it?"

"I'm a volunteer buddy with the Charbonne Clinic. We take care of AIDS patients. I'm doing it because it's important. I don't have anything important in my life anymore. Except you."

Catherine frowned. "Maybe," she said at last, "I'll come with you. If you think it would be all right."

"I'd be so pleased—"

"I'm not doing it to please you. Don't think everything's okay between us, because it isn't."

"I've got forgiving of my own to do," he said. "You've treated me like shit."

"I don't like it when you swear like that."

"Too fucking bad."

He heard her breathing.

"You're different than you used to be," she said.

"I've learned a lot. Especially tonight." He laughed. "I didn't know a lot of what I told you tonight until I told you."

"You shouldn't be proud of anything you told me."

"I'm pleased that I'm beginning to understand things."

"I don't like what I understand," she said. "I don't like being here."

"I let you down. Now you have to decide what you're going to do about it."

"What are you going to do if I write you off?"

"You already have," he said. "And I survived it. You can't trade me in or change your ancestry or begin again. I'm the only father you'll ever have."

"We'll see about that."

"Guess we will."

Things had changed. She was here safe with him. He remembered lying on her little bed in the dark, holding her while she sniffled past her nightmares. He felt her snug in his arms in the twilight on the patio, sliding into sleep.

"Good night, Catherine." He pondered the wisdom of telling her he loved her. What would he do if she didn't respond? "I love you."

"Good night," she said.

He huffed to himself. That hurt. He'd try again. And again. Parents were such patsies.

◆ ◆ ◆

The alarm rang at five. They rose, haggard and bleary. She made coffee while he showered, and they left for Peter's apartment without breakfast.

The VW's tires sang on the wet pavement in the silence

between them.

"I'm sorry about today," he said. "If only I'd known you were going to be with me—"

"I'm not here because I want to be. I don't have—"

" . . . any place else to go," he said with her in a chorus, nodding rhythmically. "I'm sorry about that, too." The street lights sailed slowly by, ringed with halos of mist. "I'm sorry your mother let you down." He bit his lip. "I'm sorry I let you down." No answer. "I'm sorry. Really. I am. I'd like to make it up to you."

"Stop saying you're sorry all the time, for God's sake. Why are you always sorry about everything?"

Martin started to speak but caught himself in time. He laughed. "I was about to say I was sorry for being sorry."

"I believe it."

He wanted to apologize again but was afraid to.

"Tell me about this man you're taking care of," Catherine said.

"Don't be scared. Peter's a person like everyone else."

"What does he look like?"

"He's very thin, and he has lesions on his face."

"Like sores or something?"

"Like somebody beat him up real bad."

"They're from the disease?"

"They're from one of the diseases. He has a bunch."

She raised and lowered her shoulders. "Don't expect me to be very cheerful or friendly."

Martin snapped on the windshield wipers. They groaned and scraped.

"Does Peter know anything about me?" she said.

"A little. He and I spend a lot of time talking. It's about all he can do."

Catherine surveyed the sky through the windshield. "How old is he?"

"Thirty-one."

"I thought he was older."

"AIDS specializes in young, gay men."

"He's gay?"

"Very. Kind of swishy."

She grimaced. "I hope I like him all right."

"You will. I know you'll like his girl friend, Sally."

"Girl friend?"

"Kind of hard to explain. And you'll like Bruce, one of his former . . . lovers."

She shifted her weight in the seat. "This is beginning to sound bizarre."

Martin scratched behind his ear. "Comes with the territory."

"What territory?"

"Life's bizarre."

"Goddam," she said in a whisper. "I never thought I'd be in a situation like this."

Martin permitted himself a small grin. "I don't like it when you swear like that."

"I was praying. I don't swear."

"Maybe I can't tell the difference."

"Maybe you can't," she said.

When Martin unlocked the door to the apartment, the desk light was on. Peter was sitting up in bed, his robe on, face washed, and hair carefully combed so that a ringlet hung over his forehead.

Martin sat next to the bed. "Morning, bunkie. What are you doing awake? You know what time it is?"

"It's going to be a special day. I don't want to waste any of it."

"How are you?"

"I slept like a mummy in an undiscovered tomb, so I'm all grins and giggles this morning. Cohen would say it's the psychological reaction of having something to look forward to. Privately, he'd tell you that hope is all-important in terminal cases. 'Gotta keep their hopes up.'"

"Peter, don't be catty."

"I know what's going on, that's all." He peered past Martin through the dark. Alarm showed in his face. "Who's with you?"

"My daughter, Catherine. Hope you don't mind. Came up sort of suddenly last night." He put out his hand toward Catherine. She approached the bed, a polite smile over her fear.

"Catherine." Peter offered her his hand.

She took it. Her eyes grazed the lesions on his knuckles. "Glad to know you."

"Can't tell you how pleased I am to know you. I think you are very brave."

"No, I . . ." She turned to Martin for help.

"Hungry?" Martin asked him.

"No."

"Good. I'll fix a big breakfast."

Martin dropped *The Washington Post* on the bed and took off his coat.

Catherine, following his lead, peeled off her coat and reached for his. "Where should I put these?"

"Closet inside the door," Peter said.

While she was hanging up their coats, Martin leaned over

the bed. "I've never *seen* such a brazen attempt at charm. You keep your hands to yourself today, young man."

"I do it well, don't I? Could have been quite a ladies' man if I hadn't had other interests, so to speak."

"So to speak."

Peter put his hands behind his head. "You're not doing too well in that department. I'll give you some pointers."

"I'll take all the help I can get." Martin folded his arms. "This is weird."

"Ain't it the truth. Now you *know* it's going to be a good day. Catherine," he said in a normal voice. "Why don't you turn on some lights? Let's cheer the place up. And how about music? Put Strauss waltzes on the stereo. Later we can all dance."

Martin and Catherine went to work. When the turkey was in the oven, the Taylor New York champagne in the refrigerator, and five stemmed glasses in the freezing compartment, Martin made breakfast for the three of them. He and Catherine sat next to the bed, breakfast plates in hand.

Martin frowned at Peter. "Eat. It'll probably hurt, but you need the nourishment."

Peter ate two bites of scrambled eggs and a sliver of bacon, put his plate aside, and leaned back on the pillows, his face tense. "I'll eat more later."

After breakfast, Martin shaved Peter, then walked him to the bathroom to brush his teeth. Martin squinted into the oven, frowned at the rising rolls on the counter, and followed Peter to the bathroom to bathe him.

"You can peel potatoes," he told Catherine over his shoulder. He stopped. "If you don't mind."

"I don't mind."

By mid-morning, Martin had the dinner well in hand. He

and Catherine moved the dining room table close to Peter's bed and covered it with a white table cloth borrowed from the Wheaton house. Martin dusted again while Catherine set the table for four and arranged a place setting on a tray. Martin set out the Nuits-Saint-Georges in the living room, away from the heat of the oven, to be opened an hour before dinner. He turned to Peter to announce that everything was progressing, but Peter had drifted off. Martin signaled Catherine to let him sleep, motioned to the desk chair, recovered *The Washington Post* from the bed, and handed it to her. He settled himself in the wing chair. Not enough sleep last night. He was already tired. He let himself go, dozed.

He woke slowly, serenely. He let his eyes stay closed while he listened to the labored breathing from the bed and an occasional rattle of newspaper from the desk chair.

He wondered at his foolish happiness. He decided to enjoy it and make it last as long as he could. He was here with the two people he loved most. Catherine hadn't forgiven him, and Peter would die soon. But they were both here now. When love was more important than anything else, people could create incandescent moments. Really powerful or really loving people could create whole hours that cast shadows backward and forward in time. He himself hadn't done it often, but he knew the possibility lay in his hands.

Why didn't he always create perfect times? Because he had forgotten what was important. Maybe the proximity of death was making him stop caring about how well he was competing, whether his income would be greater this year, or whether he was attractive. He was overcome by the urge to reach out and hold onto people he loved. He knew he might not be able to do it much longer. *Why don't we understand,* he said to himself, acknowledging the pain under his happiness, *that death is always near?*

Never mind, never mind. Tomorrow or the next day would hurt. Not today. *I'll love them. The best way I know how.* He opened his eyes, got to his feet, and walked stiffly to the kitchen, his legs still asleep.

Bruce arrived promptly at three with an armful of yellow roses and caught Martin's contagious happiness. As soon as he was in the door, he hugged Martin and wished him happy Thanksgiving. When Martin introduced him to Catherine, he asked her if he could hug her, too. She consented, a little flustered. Finally, he handed the roses to Martin and went to Peter. He put his arms around him and held him, his eyes closed. Peter clung to him.

"Look what Bruce brought," Martin said.

"My God, they're gorgeous!" Peter said.

Martin carried the roses to the bed. Peter touched the blooms with his fingertips, smelled one blossom, and turned his shining eyes on Bruce.

"How did you know . . ."

" . . . that they're your favorites?" Bruce laughed. "Because you told me years ago. You don't remember anything, do you? That's not all." He reached in his coat pocket and handed Peter a small box wrapped in glossy royal blue paper with a butter yellow ribbon. Martin and Catherine came close to the bed.

"A cordless shaver!" Peter cried. "How did you know?"

"I was guessing. If you don't like it—"

"I love it."

"Sure will save me time," Martin said. "And Peter nicks and razor burn." He cocked his head at Bruce. "And now that you've given your gifts, why don't you take off your coat?"

A knock. Sally swirled into the room.

"Hugs are in order," Martin said. She put down her parcels, slipped into his arms, and kissed his cheek. "This is my daughter, Catherine," Martin said, glowing with pride.

"I didn't know you had children." Sally hugged Catherine without asking.

"And this is Bruce . . ." Martin groped for the last name.

" . . . Dushinsky," Bruce said.

"I'm Sally Murdoch."

More hugs.

"Let me take your coat," Martin said.

She allowed Martin to help her out of it, picked up her parcels, and headed for the bed. "Hello, Pete." She left her things on the desk chair and put her arms around him.

He held her and stroked her hair. "Hello, love."

She pulled back. "I brought you something." From the chair she retrieved what was obviously a record wrapped in silver paper. "Open it."

"*Der Rosenkavalier*," he whispered. "Does it have the trio on it?"

"And the presentation of the rose, too."

He held the record to his chest.

"Did you buy another copy?" she asked.

"Didn't want to hear it without you."

He leaned forward, put his hands on her shoulders, and kissed her on the forehead.

She turned to Martin. "I brought wine."

"Not Dom Perignon," Peter said.

"Yes," she said, embarrassed, "1975. I know how you like it. I wasn't sure you could drink."

"I'll taste enough to let the bubbles tickle my tongue."

"It's already cold."

"Let's serve it now," Martin said. "I have glasses chilled."

Catherine accompanied Martin into the kitchen for glasses and an ice bucket.

"Everybody treats you like you're in charge," she said in an undertone. "You're the host, cook, and maitre d'."

"The equivalent of the hostess in our old life. Things have changed."

"You really take care of him? I mean laundry and cleaning and everything?"

"Sure. What did you think?" He took the stemmed glasses from the freezing compartment and stood them on a tray.

She shrugged. "I didn't know you knew how to do all those things."

He filled the bucket with ice and put Sally's Dom Perignon into it. "You learn fast when you're living alone and don't have any money."

She lifted the tray of glasses and waited for him to take the lead. He went past her with the ice bucket and its stand. As they came into the living room, shimmering music, all strings and harps and xylophones and gleaming soprano, filled the apartment. Sally stood by the stereo.

Martin shook open a napkin, waved it in the air, and wrapped it around the bottle. He spit in both palms, rubbed his hands together, and attacked the cork. It popped with a satisfying *whup*. They poured and toasted Peter, then Peter toasted Bruce, then he toasted Sally, and finally Catherine. He was about to toast Martin when everybody except Peter ran out of champagne.

"Will you accept a poor substitute?" Martin asked.

"Substitute, substitute!" Peter said.

Martin brought out his bottle of Taylor. The toasting continued.

Peter was so much smaller than when Martin had first seen him. He seemed fragile in the bed, covered by a pajama top far too large for him. Even the most charitable among them could no longer tell him honestly that he was pleasant to look at. Worst was the pustule to the left of his nose; it had spread down over his cheekbone and partly closed the eye above it. Now he was more like a lonely, lost, mutilated little boy than the roaring young god he had been. It didn't matter.

Catherine was polite, but she hung back, uneasy, perhaps frightened. The others would think she was shy or uncomfortable around Peter. Maybe she was. Martin knew that she wished she were not here. Not with Martin. That hurt. Maybe it would always hurt. Never mind. *She's here. I love her, and she's here.*

When dinner was ready, Catherine, Bruce, Sally, and Martin seated themselves at the table next to Peter's bed.

"Somebody should say grace," Sally said.

"Let me," Peter said. They bowed their heads. Peter closed his eyes. "Thank you, oh God. You have given me wonderful food and drink, a good place to stay, a good life. Most of all, you have given me people to love. And they love me back. Can you beat that? Forgive me, if you can, the evils I've done. Bless and keep these, my friends, whom I hold most dear. Amen."

They were silent. Martin tried to say "amen," but he had no voice.

"Hey," Peter said. "It's over. Somebody say 'amen' and let's eat."

"Amen," Catherine whispered.

The dinner was a humble affair. Or so it seemed to Martin when he saw it from Catherine's point of view. The turkey was acceptable. Its tender, moist meat sliced easily with the knife brought from Wheaton. The creamed onions and peas were only a little overcooked. But the mashed potatoes tasted like paper napkins dissolved in hot water; the gravy was all lumps.

After tasting the potatoes and gravy, Sally laughed until tears streamed down her face. "Tell me, Martin," she said as she wiped her eyes. "Where *did* you get the recipe for the gravy?"

Martin raised his eyebrows. "It's French." He lifted his hand with studied elegance and examined his fingernails. "The French *always* do it that way." Catherine wouldn't laugh, but amusement flickered around her lips.

The Nuits-Saint-Georges was delicious. So were Martin's rolls and the pie and the chicory coffee. Everyone except Catherine laughed over anecdotes and quips. Listening more than talking, Peter beamed from the bed. But the food was wasted on him—he ate almost nothing.

Catherine and Sally put away the leftovers and washed dishes while Bruce wiped the table and moved it back to the alcove. Martin pulled the desk chair up next to the bed. "How're you doing, bunkie?"

"I'm very tired and very happy," Peter said. "I've had a wonderful Thanksgiving."

"How about if I tell everyone to go home so you can get some rest?"

Peter closed his eyes and nodded.

Sally volunteered to stay behind and give Peter his bath and change his sheets. Bruce agreed to stay until she was finished and drive her home.

"What time do you want to go back to the dorm

tomorrow?" Martin asked Catherine in an undertone.

"I can't get in until noon."

"How about," Martin said to Sally, "if you tell Peter I won't be here until one or so tomorrow and put out food for him for breakfast when you leave tonight?"

Sally frowned toward Peter's sleeping figure in the bed. "You think he'll be all right alone that long?"

"Leave the phone on the desk chair next to the bed. He can call me if he needs anything."

They whispered good night.

◈ ◈ ◈

Martin and Catherine drove home in what threatened to be a silent ride.

"Sorry we had so little time to ourselves," he said as if resuming a conversation.

"You treat Peter like a son," Catherine said. "Here you are, pouring love on him like it's about to overflow, but you walked out on me. I think you're all screwed up."

"Quick to pass judgment, aren't we? Live a few years before you condemn people for not doing what you want."

"Is Peter," she said with cold smile, "a substitute for *me*?"

"Part of the reason I'm taking care of Peter is that you won't let me take care of you. That's only part. I don't have a family anymore. My work is the pits. I'm alone."

"Come on. I thought you were the Don Juan of suburbia, the Casanova of the arty academic crowd."

"Stop it! You have no business talking to me like that."

She stared at the empty streets through the window.

"I had to find something to live for," he said. "I'm a failure, Catherine. I've learned from watching your mother that success ain't all it's cracked up to be. Anyway, I wanted to give something to somebody else."

Catherine turned. "It's all to make you feel better. Jeez, I feel sorry for your women. They're nothing but ego trips for you."

He swallowed. "I volunteered to take care of Peter partly to find something that would make me feel like I mattered. I love Peter now. That makes me see things I didn't see before."

"What's the difference? You still do it to feel better about yourself. You actually *enjoy* taking care of him, don't you?"

"If I believed that the best thing for Peter would be for me to get out of his life and never see him again, I'd be gone. Peter's existence makes me happy." He breathed deeply. "So does yours."

"And Mom's?"

"It did once." He was sweating. "Some of it was selfish. I wanted her to care about me. When she didn't, the world came to an end. When she didn't care about you, I wanted to kill her." He glanced at her. She was facing him. "But part of me gloried in her being alive. I never wanted to hurt her. I wanted to shock her back to reality. It didn't work. That's why I didn't fight her in the divorce." He mopped his forehead. "I gave up."

"You shouldn't have walked out and left me." Her voice quavered.

"It was the dumbest, most unforgivable thing I ever did. At the time I was so upset I wasn't thinking straight."

"I loved you, Daddy. I didn't want you to go."

Martin couldn't answer. He blinked and swallowed hard and set his teeth to endure the hurting in his chest.

Chapter 8

The Leer

Martin awoke early Friday morning. While he was folding the bed clothes, the phone rang. Sally.

"Anything wrong?" Martin said.

"I decided to sleep at Peter's last night. He's got a camping cot. I wonder if it's time for round-the-clock care. I'd be willing to help—you know, take turns staying with Peter."

"Let me check with the clinic."

After lunch, as the autumn sunshine knifed through the clouds, Martin drove Catherine to the dorm. "You can stay at my place any time."

"Craig's kind of, you know . . ."

"Might do you good to be around people like him. You're a little—forgive me for saying it—holier-than-thou."

"Not really." She pushed back her hair with both hands. "I'm not a monk, either, Daddy."

Martin blinked. "You mean you—"

"Not very much." She perked. "Surprised?"

"Guess I didn't think of you as a sexual, um, person. We have something in common."

"Both sexual people?"

"No, that we don't do it very much." Martin shook his head in wonder. "Oddest conversation I've ever had."

They drove in silence.

"Have dinner with me one night next week?" he asked as they pulled up.

"I need time to get myself together. You've given me a lot to think about."

After Sally left, Peter watched the sunshine come and go on Porter Street. Martin wouldn't help him find Johnny's mother. He was afraid an outing might make Peter sicker. Peter would have to do it by himself or get someone else to help. Maybe without Martin knowing. Sally? No way. Billy was too sick. Kirk, Joey, Ron? He didn't want their help. Bruce? Maybe.

First, though, he had to find her. What about the phone book? He'd call her. Crazy thought. What would he say to her? Wouldn't he be reminding her of Johnny's death?

Not to worry. He'd be doing it for himself, not for her, not out of goodness. "Goodness is beyond reward," but he wanted his reward—forgiveness. On the other hand, maybe if he talked to her, that would do good. A friend of Johnny's. Maybe he could say something nice and make her feel better.

He shot a glance at the telephone on the dining room chair by the bed. The thought of calling her terrified him, but he could feel his body shutting down. At the very last minute he would know that he'd wasted his life. It would be better if he had never lived. Damnation? Maybe that's what it was.

He had to try. He struggled from the bed and lugged the Northern Virginia telephone book, a pencil, and a note pad from the desk. Out of breath, he propped himself against the headboard and turned to the L's. He found two and a half columns of Logans. With a sigh, he started through them. Johnny had told Peter that his father had died years before, so the search had to be for a woman's name, or perhaps a Mrs. Man's-name Logan.

When he got to the J's, he found three Johns and—he gasped—*Johnny Logan*. On Old Dominion Boulevard in Alexandria. Could Johnny's number still be in the book? He underlined it and continued to search. In the M's, he found "Mrs. Marjorie." He checked the address and number. They were the same as Johnny's.

Jesus. Could he do this? He had to.

Trembling, he took the telephone in his lap and dialed. It rang three times and a woman answered.

Peter wondered what to say. "Mrs. Logan?"

"Yes?"

His heart pounded. "Mrs. Marjorie Logan?"

"Yes?" It was a nice voice, an alto voice, clear and free of malice. He could see her—tall, stately, calm, a handsome woman, her face at once sad and noble. "Mrs. Logan, my name is Peter Christopher. I was a friend of a man named Johnny Logan who died last March. Are you by any chance, I mean, were you—" Peter took a breath. "—his mother?"

"Yes," she answered, her voice lower, "I am Johnny's mother."

He hesitated. "I'm calling to tell you how sorry I was about Johnny."

Silence. Peter tightened.

"Thank you, Peter. May I call you Peter?"

"Of course. Johnny was a fine person. And a good friend. We all miss him."

"So many people have said so. It's a comfort."

"I was especially concerned because, well, I have AIDS, too."

"Peter," she said, distressed. "I'm so sorry."

"I'm being taken care of."

"Can I do anything?"

Peter was abashed. She was offering to help him?

"Are you at Lincoln College?" she asked.

"No, I . . ." He gnawed his lip. "I met Johnny through mutual friends."

"Sorry I didn't recognize your name."

"I don't think we ever met." Unless she hung out in gay bars. A gay groupie, a fruit fly. Peter was instantly ashamed.

"You never came to the house?" she said. "Johnny had so many friends."

"No, I never did."

"It would be such a pleasure to meet you."

He clutched. Meet her? Face to face?

"Maybe you could drop by for coffee," she said.

"I don't get out much. Maybe some time during one of my good spells." What if he invited her to come and see him. Screwy notion.

"I'm home evenings and weekends," she said. "You caught me here today because schools are closed on the Friday after Thanksgiving. I'm a teacher. Give me a call any time and drop over."

"That's so nice of you."

"Thank you for calling, Peter. I'm pleased that you cared enough. Most people are afraid they'll make things worse. It helps me to talk to people who knew him."

Peter swallowed. "I'm sorry I didn't do it before. I guess I was a little scared."

"That's kind of you. Do come and see me."

He hung up. He did it. He called Johnny's mother.

"Hello," Martin said.

Peter jumped. He hadn't heard him come in.

Martin dropped *The Washington Post* on the coffee table by the bed. "Who were you talking to?"

"Just someone."

"Had lunch?"

"Sal left some stuff. I wasn't hungry."

"Relax. I'll fix something."

Peter barely touched his food. Martin frowned. "Mouth, throat, or stomach?"

"All three."

"What would taste good? What wouldn't hurt?"

"This tastes good. Nothing would be better."

Martin looked defeated. "We'll ask Cohen."

"Yes," Peter echoed sardonically, "we always ask Cohen."

Martin took his plate.

"I shaved myself," Peter said. "See?"

"You missed a spot." Martin poked Peter's jaw.

"I didn't have a mirror." Peter rubbed his cheek. "You'd think the hair would stop growing when other functions of the body stop working. I read somewhere that hair and fingernails on corpses go on growing." He watched the sky through the window. "I'm really in a funny mood today. You know, I think Bruce and Sally gave me those things as, like, early Christmas presents. I think they're afraid I won't make it to Christmas. You think I'll make it to Christmas?"

"I don't know."

"Please tell me."

"I really don't know, Peter."

"I've lost a lot of ground lately. And I'm gruesome, aren't I?"

"Not to me. That's because I know you and . . . love you."

Love me? First time Martin had said that. *Let it go for now. It'll get in the way.* "What did Catherine say? Did I scare her?"

"She had to get used to you."

"Because I look gruesome, right?"

Martin paused. "From her perspective, you probably do."

Peter heaved a sigh of satisfaction. "Thank you. I knew you'd tell me the truth. You're a brave man, Martin. Catherine is a wonderful person. Did you two make up?"

"No. Her mother stood her up."

"So she's still mad at you?"

"I don't know." Martin grimaced. "She thinks I abandoned her."

"I wish I could do something."

Martin's face eased. "Thanks. Nothing you can do."

"Sometimes help comes from unlikely places."

Martin shook his head.

"I wish you'd talk to me more about important things," Peter said. "You hardly ever say anything about yourself. I'm a good listener, you know. Had a talk with Sally last night. Told her how I felt about her. Should have told her not to give me early Christmas presents, though."

"What do you want to do at Christmas?"

"Have some people in, if I'm up to it and if you're willing. Only at Christmas, I'd like my mom and dad to be here." He grinned. "Surprised?"

Martin blanched. "When did you decide this?"

"Middle of the night. Got to thinking about Christmas and how my mom would be asking me to come home and I'd have to lie. I forgot to tell you. I called yesterday while you and Catherine were doing the laundry. Told Mom we wouldn't be coming for dinner."

"My God. What was your excuse?"

"Made something up," Peter said with a wave of his hand.

"Peter, what did you tell her?"

"Said I got a call to do a banquet at the Cosmos Club—a request I couldn't refuse."

"Peter!" Martin shook his head.

"And I told her you went out the night before and got snockered and were in no shape to appear."

Martin's mouth dropped open.

"That was the gist of it," Peter said. "Colored the story up a little to make it sound plausible. Something about an old girlfriend who was on uppers and kept pouring you gin on the rocks."

"*Peter!*"

"Had to be a good story. Otherwise she wouldn't have believed it. If she caught me lying, she'd have *really* been mad."

"She wasn't mad at that version of events?"

"Furious. Livid. Could have killed us both."

"Jesus," Martin said. "What she must think of me!"

"One of the principles of successful lying is to make the story so outlandish and embarrassing that nobody would ever believe you made it up."

"Peter," Martin said, now genuinely irritated, "you are a real asshole."

Peter held up his hand, palm outward. "Please. Don't use the word 'asshole' in vain. Where I come from, it's a term of endearment."

Martin snarled in wordless frustration. "And you want to have them here for Christmas? I don't think I could ever face them after that story."

"By then they'll know the truth. I want you to go see them.

Tell them I'm gay. Tell them I have AIDS. Prepare them for how I look."

Martin closed his eyes and shook his head as if to clear out the shock waves. "Jesus Christ. I don't know. Let me think about it."

"There's no hurry." Peter rubbed the corner of his eye with his index finger. "Thank you for telling me you love me. I knew it, but I've been waiting for you to say it."

After lunch, while Martin went about his chores, Peter lay with his eyes closed, but his mind was working. Maybe he could do something really good after all. Something for someone else. Maybe he could help Martin. What would it take to get Catherine to forgive Martin? What if Peter talked to her—on the sly, of course? Was there any way he could show her about forgiveness?

A thought flashed. What if Catherine went with him to see Mrs. Logan? What if Catherine actually saw forgiveness in practice—for something far worse than Martin had ever dreamed of doing? Peter gave his head a fast shake. What was he fantasizing about this time? Maybe the virus was scrambling his brain. He wasn't even sure he could face Mrs. Logan. And how could he get Catherine to go? Martin wouldn't even *think* of letting her go. Somehow he'd have to slip out with Catherine without Martin knowing. Insane. Forget it.

But what a lovely idea.

Martin changed Peter's soiled bed and put clean sheets on the cot while Peter made his way to the bathroom to brush his teeth. Martin gathered the lunch dishes and washed them. He pictured himself in the Christophers' living room somewhere in one of the more fashionable neighborhoods of Baltimore, seated on a peach-and-coral-period pink sofa, quietly sipping gin and explaining calmly to Roger and Alicia that Peter was gay, had AIDS, and was dying. Oh, and that he looked gruesome.

He rinsed the last cup, put it in the drainer, and washed the dish pan. He imagined meeting Roger and Alicia in a quiet restaurant. He'd explain Peter's condition over cocktails. Perhaps he'd have a snapshot with him to show them so that they wouldn't be too horrified when they saw him. Or maybe he and Roger would do lunch and Roger could explain it all to Alicia. No, he thought as he took his gloves off and tied up the garbage bag, no, that would never do.

"I'm taking the garbage down," he called to Peter.

Negative fantasies bounced around in Martin's head as he vacuumed, got the mail from the lobby, and cleaned the bathroom. He considered and rejected one scenario after another. While Peter soaked in the tub, Martin called the clinic's AIDS Services Coordinator and asked for help with twenty-four-hour care for Peter. The coordinator promised to get right on it. Martin changed Peter's bed again when he found it damp with sweat and got Peter into fresh pajamas and back in bed. Finally, before heading into the kitchen to finish the shopping list, he drew up the desk chair next to the bed.

"Peter," he said, "if it was a decent thing to do, I'd talk to your parents. It's not. They have a right to hear the truth from you."

"Okay," Peter said. "I'll ask somebody else."

"Why don't *you* tell them?"

Peter lay on his side, his back to Martin. With a sigh, Martin rose and went to the kitchen.

Peter was silent and distant the rest of the afternoon. Late in the day, Martin shopped for groceries and returned to find Peter asleep, so he worked at the dining room table on his students' harmony assignments. At dusk, Peter awoke with a spasm of coughing.

Martin frowned. "Your cough is getting worse."

"Have to tell Cohen," Peter rasped.

"What do you want for dinner?"

Peter rolled on his side facing Martin. "I'm not hungry."

"Have something anyway. What was your weight the last time you saw Cohen?"

"A hundred-twenty-four and sliding."

"Better eat something."

"I don't think I can." Peter turned on his back and stared at the ceiling. "Martin, I'm sorry I was pissed at you. I don't want to be mad at you anymore. At least I got to the point of knowing they have to be told. That's something, isn't it?"

"That's a lot, bunkie."

"I'm feelin' mighty peaked. Would you hold me a while?"

Martin took off his shoes, sat on the bed, and leaned against the headboard. Peter rested his head against Martin's chest. Martin held him and felt his ragged breathing. Soon Peter was asleep.

Peter awoke certain he'd figured out how to sneak out, see Mrs. Logan, and take Catherine with him. All he had to do was con Bruce into picking up Catherine and driving them to Mrs. Logan's. The whole idea was so outrageous, so fiendishly clever. Peter was awed by his own creativity.

Martin was talking on the telephone. Peter lay with his eyes closed and listened. "Eight? Fine. I'll be back in the morning and plan to stay here tomorrow night." He hung up.

Peter stretched and opened his eyes.

"That was Sally," Martin said. "She'll be spending the night." Martin gave him an apologetic smile. "We've decided you shouldn't be left alone. I'm trying to arrange around-the-clock care for you from the clinic. Meanwhile, Sally and I—"

"What am I? Chopped *pâté de foie gras*? Doesn't anybody think they should consult me before they make plans for me? I feel like Alice hearing the talk about sending her by post."

Martin colored.

"You poor innocent," Peter said. "So little dawns on you."

Martin frowned at the floor.

Peter touched Martin's hand. "It's all right. You're only doing what's best for me. I'm sorry I snapped. I don't like it when people take control of my life away from me."

"You're right."

Peter stretched his arm as if pushing something from him and appraised his fingernails through hooded eyes. "I'll let it go this time. As long as you don't try to fix me up with any of your old girlfriends. What's for dinner?"

Bruce called at seven and asked if he could drop by. His visit was brief.

"I have a very special favor to ask of you, Bruce," Peter whispered while Martin was in the kitchen. "I want you to drive me somewhere. I'm going to ask Catherine James, Martin's daughter, to go with us. This Sunday if I can arrange it. Martin won't be here then. Sally will be taking care of me."

Bruce's perennial smile weakened. "Why not ask Martin or Sally to take you?"

"They'd never let me go. They think I'm too sick."

"Then maybe you shouldn't do it, Peter."

"I have to. It's so important that even if it shortens my life, I'll do it. I want to visit a woman whose son died of AIDS. Martin and Sally don't understand, but I know you do."

Bruce scowled. "Well . . ."

"Thank you, Bruce. You're a love. Would you mind picking up Catherine at Morton Hall on the GW campus at 12:30 on Sunday and bringing her over here?"

Bruce nodded uncertainly.

Bruce had just left when Sally arrived. Martin gave her a hug, asked her to check Peter over, and went to say good night to him.

"Hope things get better with Catherine," Peter said.

"Let me worry about it," Martin said.

When Martin was gone, Sally put on latex gloves, pulled back Peter's covers, and unbuttoned his pajama top.

"Don't be fresh," he said.

She felt his neck with both hands, her face serious.

"You're going to have to practice your leer," Peter said. He licked his lips. "Your seduction techniques have slipped."

"Shut up, Pete."

"Want me to take off my pants?"

"Pete, cut it out."

She felt his stomach, pressed with her fingertips on his sides, put her ear to his chest, and listened.

"What's your prognosis?" Peter asked.

"Don't know. You're about the same."

"Martin didn't do the laundry, Sally," Peter said, all innocence. "Would you mind?"

"Of course not."

He waited for Sally to leave with the laundry, then took the phone in his lap. First he called Catherine. "Don't have but a minute to talk, and I want to ask you to help me."

"Certainly, Peter," she said, surprise in her voice. "You all right?"

"I'm lousy, but that's not what I want to talk about." He explained that he wanted to visit someone in Alexandria. Bruce would pick her up on Sunday. "Will you go with me, Catherine? I know it's a lot to ask."

Catherine was silent for a moment. "This is all so sudden. How did you get my number?"

"Filched it from your father's pocket while he was taking the garbage out."

"He doesn't know?"

"No, and I'd appreciate it if you didn't tell him. He wouldn't let me go."

"Peter, do you, like, get out?"

Peter laughed. "Of course. Why not?" He took a deep breath. "This visit is very important to me."

"Why are you asking me?"

"I guessed that you'd help me. Not everybody would." He congratulated himself on his slickness. "You'll help me?"

She hesitated. "I hope it's okay. Who do you want to visit?"

"A woman whose son died of AIDS. I knew him."

"I see."

"So I can count on you for Sunday?"

"I guess so."

"Wonderful. Thanks so much. Got to go now."

Next, trembling, he dialed Marjorie Logan's number. Yes, she said, she would be home between one and two on Sunday, and she would love to see him. Last, he left a message on Bruce's answering machine confirming the plan.

"What would have to happen," Peter asked Martin over dinner Saturday night, "for Catherine to forgive you?"

Martin straightened in surprise. "Maybe when she grows up, when she sees that people are people, that they make mistakes. Why?"

"I've been thinking about forgiveness lately. I need a lot of that myself. And I wish my parents would forgive me."

"You could start by forgiving them."

"I'm trying."

At eleven the following morning, after Martin had left, Peter called to Sally in the kitchen. "I need a bath, Sally. Would you mind?"

"I'll fill the tub."

When he was clean and dry, he combed his hair, feeling his way, wishing he had a mirror. Sally brought him fresh pajamas.

"I want to put on real clothes today," he said.

"You must be feeling better."

"I am," he lied.

She helped him into plaid slacks, a white dress shirt, and a blue sweater. He sat before the television, giddy with weakness. While Sally was in the bathroom, he took twenty dollars from the cigar box, found his keys, and copied Mrs. Logan's address onto a slip of paper.

He timed his request for lunch just right. As soon as he finished, Sally would wash his dishes, tie up the trash, and take it to the basement. He dallied over his soup and French bread but forced himself to eat all of it. At twelve-thirty, he sopped up the last dollop, leaned back, and rubbed his belly. At quarter to one, right on schedule, Sally told him she was taking the garbage down. He glanced up from the television, smiled, nodded, and returned his eyes to the screen.

As soon as her steps receded down the hall, he was on his feet. He scribbled a note saying that he had to do something very important and would be back soon. "Don't worry about me." He was out the door and floundered down the hall.

He prayed that the elevator would be empty. It was. He descended to the lobby level, swallowing the urge to vomit, and walked slowly, evenly. He averted his eyes to avoid the wall mirror behind the desk clerk's counter. Finally, he was out the glass doors.

The circular driveway beyond the portico was empty. What if there had been a hitch? What if Bruce or Catherine telephoned to say they were late? What if Sally—who would undoubtedly search for him immediately—found him here before they arrived? He chewed his nails in the pale sunshine and buttoned his car coat. He wished he could sit down. He was trembling. Colors were vivid, textures grainy, movements blurred.

An electric blue Maxima sped up the drive and came to a sudden stop in front of him. Bruce leapt from the driver's side, his face dark, his overcoat so green that Peter was mesmerized.

"What the fuck are you doing out here?" Bruce said. "I was going to come up and get you."

Catherine emerged from the car like a visitation in a flowing slate-colored coat and blood-red scarf decorated with bold, black cursive Chinese characters. Peter squinted at them. He shut his eyes and shook his head. His brain tingled. When he focused again, her face—serious, concerned—was close to his. He could see the pores on her nose.

"Peter," she said, "are you all right?"

"Fine, fine," he laughed. "What's all the commotion?" He handed Bruce Mrs. Logan's address. "Come on, let's go."

They bundled him into the back seat and fretted aloud about the cold and the wind. As they pulled away, he closed his eyes and heaved a sigh, partly of relief, partly of exhaustion. As they cleared the circular drive and headed back down Quebec Street toward Connecticut Avenue, Peter scanned the entrance to the building. Sally swept through the doors. She peered in all directions. He slid down in the seat, sure she hadn't seen him. Despite the shakes he hid, despite the alarms going off all over his body, Peter giggled to himself. It was fun.

As he drove, Bruce lectured Peter on allowing his friends to take care of him properly. Catherine said nothing. She occasionally twisted her neck toward him as if to assure herself that he hadn't died. Each time she did, her red and black scarf hypnotized him. He smiled genially at her. She frowned and turned back to the front.

They drove south on Connecticut to Pennsylvania, left past the White House, right toward the 14th Street Bridge. After they crossed the Potomac, Bruce drove in silence and glowered at the exit signs on Route 395. Peter caught snatches of his own reflection in the rearview mirror and the side mirrors and instantly slammed his eyes shut.

Bruce was handsome and elfish and macho all at the same time. He drove confidently, in command, with swagger. Peter hadn't swaggered in a long, long time, but he knew what it felt like. He was glad Bruce could still do it.

Peter dozed. When the car stopped, he jolted awake.

"We're here," Bruce said.

They were on a tree-lined road that curved upward on a hill. Sedate little houses in brick and white trim were everywhere, each decked out with its own narrow driveway, patch of lawn, and clutch of shrubs. The houses stood lifeless in the cold sunshine. The street was deserted.

Peter shook off the last webs of sleep. "Which house?"

"That one," Bruce said.

"Would you mind waiting in the car, Bruce?"

"If that's what you want."

"Catherine, help me."

She hurried from the front seat and opened his door. He leaned on her as he got from the car, stood for a moment, and gathered his senses.

"Let's go."

Refusing himself the luxury of tottering, he pushed her hand away and strutted up the walk, up the six steps to the porch. He steeled himself against a rush of dizziness and rang the bell.

The door opened. Before them stood a stout, aging woman in an ample blue print dress, her short hair wavy and white with blue undertones. She looked up at Peter. Her lips parted as her blue eyes explored his. The revulsion in her face was unmistakable. She closed her mouth. "Peter Christopher."

"Yes," Peter said, out of breath.

"I'm Marjorie Logan. Come in, come in. Let me take your coats."

Peter and Catherine followed her into the house. They turned left past a murky, cramped stairway, into a tiny living room filled with lace, dark wood, old photographs, and musty smells. Peter halted when he saw his book of Chinese writings on the coffee table. Johnny peered into his eyes from a large black-and- white photograph on the upright piano. The face was younger than Peter had remembered, but the grin was immediately recognizable. Peter's pulse raced.

"Sit down, sit down," Mrs. Logan said. "Can I get you anything? I have fresh date nut bread I baked this morning. And maybe coffee?"

"Nothing for me," Peter said. "By the way, I'd like you to meet Catherine James."

"How about you, Catherine?" Mrs. Logan said. "What can I get you?"

"I'd love coffee and some of your bread."

Mrs. Logan scurried away. Peter gazed at the picture. Johnny's clear, untroubled eyes looked straight into Peter's, as if the world were at peace and there were nothing to fear. Abruptly, Mrs. Logan's hulk blocked Peter's view.

"Here you are." She offered Catherine a cup and a plate and cleared space on the coffee table, shoving aside red and green construction paper stars, bells, trees, and sleds. "Doodads from my first-graders."

Catherine nibbled. "Lovely cake."

"Old recipe," Mrs. Logan said as she sat heavily in an ancient rocking chair opposite them. "My mother always made it for the holidays when she could get the ingredients. That wasn't always possible on a farm in West Virginia. We didn't even have running water and electricity until I was six. Of course, nowadays . . . Listen to me run on. Comes from spending so much time alone." She turned to Peter. "Since Johnny died, I don't socialize. So nice to talk to someone who knew him."

"Are you doing okay, Mrs. Logan?" Peter said.

"I get by." She rocked gently. Her face wrinkled and her eyes watered. "It's not the same without him, of course. I miss him so much sometimes, I don't know what I'll do." She laughed. "Johnny was the most important thing in my life. I married late and never expected to have children. When Johnny came along, I . . ." She put her hand to her mouth. "I get by."

"Did you like his music?" Peter said.

"I must confess," she said with embarrassment. "I don't understand it. I've got tapes he made, and I've played through his manuscripts at the piano. I'm afraid it's beyond me. Are you a musician, Peter?"

"No. I am . . . was a dancer."

"Where did you and Johnny meet?"

Peter let his eyes wander. Tell her the truth? "At the Back Door."

She wrinkled her brow.

"A bar," he said. "On an alley near P Street in D.C."

She faltered. He felt Catherine stiffen.

"It's a gay bar, Mrs. Logan."

Her face was severe. "I didn't know he went to bars."

"I saw him there three or four times before we . . ." He didn't know how to say it.

She turned her head toward the hall as if startled by a sound. Catherine, trying to steady herself, reached for her coffee. Peter leaned forward.

"I'm sorry," Peter said. "I didn't mean to shock you. Please don't be angry. You asked on the phone if you could do anything for me. You can. If you don't mind my being direct."

"What can I do?"

"Tell me stuff."

"I don't know—"

"Like, did you know Johnny was gay?"

She raised her chin and fixed Peter with her eyes. "I knew. It hurt at first. I sort of got used to the idea. He was secretive. I worried about him. I was afraid he'd get hooked up with bad people."

"Did you ever, you know, forgive him?"

Mrs. Logan frowned.

"For getting AIDS, I mean," Peter said. "And for being gay?"

Mrs. Logan gave Peter such a harsh look that he thought she wasn't going to answer. "Peter, Johnny was my boy. I loved him. There was nothing to forgive."

Peter examined his fingernails. "I know I'm asking things I have no right to ask, Mrs. Logan, but I don't have much time." He drew a careful breath. "Did he ever mention me?"

"Not that I recall. He talked about this one and that one, different friends he had. I had the feeling I never heard about the men he . . ." She stopped. "Some people I'd never met came to the funeral. They were very nice to me. I never knew how they were connected with Johnny. I made guesses about that, too." She pulled a tissue from her sleeve and brushed her nose. "I thought maybe one of them gave Johnny the disease."

"It wasn't any of them, Mrs. Logan," Peter said in a monotone.

Catherine paused in mid-sip and fixed her eyes on him.

"How . . ." Mrs. Logan said.

He swallowed hard. "It was me."

Mrs. Logan stared at Peter. Her hands tightened on the rocker's armrests until her knuckles bulged.

"I knew I had it," Peter said. "I didn't tell him. He needed to be careful. I knew what I was doing. He didn't. I didn't mean to hurt him, Mrs. Logan. I'm sorrier about Johnny than I have ever been about anything in my life."

Catherine, trembling, set her cup on the coffee table. Mrs. Logan showed no sign of breathing.

Peter lowered his eyes. "I came here to tell you what I did to Johnny and to you. Johnny was a good man. A sweet kid, really. I wasn't. There's no excuse for me. I don't want to die with Johnny's death on my conscience. I don't know what to do.

So I came to you. I have no right to tell you all this and hurt you even more. I have to. I have no right to ask you, but I will anyway."

Dizziness swept over him.

"Mrs. Logan, I'd ask Johnny to forgive me, but he can't. He's dead." He fought off a wave of trembling. "Will you forgive me?"

He let his eyes rest on her dark, worn carpet. No sound came from her. He wiped his nose with the back of his hand. Finally, he lifted his head.

Mrs. Logan was glaring toward the hall as if listening to something he couldn't hear. She lifted her hand and bit the knuckle of her index finger. Her face was a web of wrinkles. Now her red eyes flooded him with revulsion, pain, and hatred.

"Please say something," he said.

She closed her mouth and smoothed her skirt. Her throat cleared. She wiped at her nose with her tissue. "I knew someone had infected him, but I never dreamed . . ." She shook her head. "I want you to go away," she said, her voice grinding. "I don't want you in my house. I'm sorry. I'm a Christian woman, and I want to be kind. But not to you." She stood, no longer heavy and tired, full of strength. "Please go away."

"Mrs. Logan," Peter began.

"Now," she said with more force.

He opened his mouth to plead, but her face stopped him. Hatred poured from her. Her breasts rose and fell between arms tensed as if to strike. *She wants to see me dead. She'll never forgive me.*

It couldn't end like this. She was his last hope.

His trembling ceased. Cold embraced him. The dizziness disappeared. His breathing slowed to nothing. His body was calm, his mind silent. He felt a mocking smile widen his mouth. "Yes, I will go away." He laughed. Mrs. Logan shuddered. He turned to Catherine, sitting stricken beside him. "Come, Catherine." His leer grew. "Mrs. Logan has asked us to leave."

Catherine stumbled to her feet and followed him to the door. Mrs. Logan didn't move. They took their coats, left the house, and went down the steps to the walk. Peter couldn't feel his legs or feet. He was floating. Catherine grabbed his arm and propelled him forward. The horizon shifted. The car, the trees, the shrubs, the little driveways, the little houses—everything jittered. His brain was buzzing. Catherine got him into the car.

"That didn't take long," Bruce said. His voice reverberated.

Peter laughed again. "No, it didn't."

"What's wrong?" Bruce said. "Did something happen?"

Catherine began to cry.

Wearier than he could ever recall, Peter leaned back against the seat. His mind darted through options. No medicine he had was sure to kill. He had no gun. Could he get to the roof of his building? There were kitchen knives. Could he be sure if he slit his wrists?

Chapter 9

Learning to Boogie

Martin knelt on Peter's bed and grimaced through the window. In the anemic sunshine, naked trees cast skeleton shadows on the pavement of Porter Street. Foolish to hope Peter would come marching up the hill from the park to the back of the apartment building. Anything was better than sitting and trying for the hundredth time to figure out where he'd gone.

Martin slid from the bed and slumped in the desk chair. "We could go through his address book and call every number."

"I've been all over the desk hunting for it," Sally said from the wing chair, massaging her hands. "No dice. There's a locked box in the bottom bureau drawer. I think he used to keep it in there."

"No key?"

She held out her hands, palms up, and shrugged.

Martin scratched behind both ears. "Let's go over it again. Did he mention anybody?"

She shook her head.

"Talk about any place like a restaurant or bar or anything?"

"No. He was quieter than usual. Cheerful. Considerate. Cooperative. I should have realized I was being set up."

"We know he's not at Cunniption's or the Cock Pit or the Long Horn or the Back Door or Billy's. They'll call if he shows up. Cohen hasn't heard from him. He's not at the Riche. He could be in the park. We could easily have driven right by him."

"Maybe," Sally said, "it's time to call his parents."

"God, I hate to do that."

"They might know something—be able to suggest a place to search."

"I doubt it. They know nothing about Peter's life. I can't imagine Peter going to see them. And I know he wouldn't want me to call them."

For a long time, neither spoke. The gloom deepened as the light from the window dwindled.

Sally got to her feet. "I can't sit any more. How about some tea?"

A confusion of footfalls on carpet outside the door. Martin stood. Muffled voices. A scrape, a thud against the door, then a demanding knock. Martin dashed to the door, yanked it open. Three silhouettes, like cupolas of a Russian church, the highest in the middle.

"Help us get him in." Bruce's voice. The figure to Martin's left. The tall one was Peter. The short one on the right was . . .

"Catherine!"

Sally shot past Martin in a blur. She took Peter's arm from Catherine's shoulder and put it over her own. She and Bruce walked Peter to the bed. Martin gawked at Catherine in the doorway.

"Help me get his clothes off," Sally said. "Is he chilled?"

"No," Bruce said. "Just acting very strange."

"Martin," Sally said, "bring water."

"Come in and close the door," Martin said to Catherine in a hoarse whisper. He ran to the kitchen, filled a glass, brought it to the bed.

Sally snatched it. "Make tea. Add honey and lemon juice."

She sat on the bed and propped Peter against her. "Drink."

Catherine was already in the kitchen filling the kettle.

Martin set the tea pot on the counter. "Fill it with hot tap water so that the tea will stay warm longer." He lit a burner with a match. She slid the kettle onto the flame and filled the pot.

"He's sweating like a lawn sprinkler," Sally said in the living room.

"Want me to draw a tub of water?" Bruce said.

"No, let's get him comfortable. Bring towels. And pajamas. In the bureau."

Footsteps to the bathroom. Drawer opening and closing. "Will these do?"

"We should be wearing latex gloves," Sally said. "Fine time to think of it. They're in the bathroom. Top of the commode."

Martin tried to speak, failed, tried again. "What—"

"He wanted to visit someone," Catherine said in a jittery voice. "Mrs. Logan."

"Johnny's mother?"

She nodded. "He asked her to forgive him."

Martin snapped his eyes shut. Of course. Why hadn't he thought of Mrs. Logan? "How did you—"

"He called me. Told me not to tell you. Said you wouldn't let him go."

He tipped his head toward the living room. "Do you see why?"

She nodded.

"Why you?" he said.

She shrugged.

"Why didn't you tell me?" Martin said.

"He told me not to."

"That's all it took?"

"He said it was very important." She raised her eyes. "Turned out it was. He was responsible for her son's death."

"He wanted her to forgive him?"

"She didn't. She told us to leave."

"Peter," Sally's voice said, "how do you feel?"

No sound.

"Peter, what is it?" Sally said.

No answer.

"Is he conscious?" Bruce said.

"Yes. It's not that. Peter, what happened?"

No answer.

"After the dust settles," Martin said softly, "we'll talk this through, but right now, promise me you'll never do anything with Peter again without telling me."

Catherine nodded.

When and how? No weapons. He didn't even own a carving knife. No razors. No poisons. None of his windows opened. The grating irony was that Billy had been right. He should have done it as soon as he was diagnosed and saved himself all this. Maybe the way Billy planned. Calvert Street Bridge. He could go by cab. No, they'd stop him. From now on, they'd watch him.

He could still feel the burn of Mrs. Logan's eyes. Her body, focused with hate, her chest heaving. He'd done the unforgivable because he *was* the unforgivable. She wanted him dead. So did he.

All he could see was the red inside his eyelids shot with bolts of anguish. God's mistake. His hands squirmed with the desire to tear the flesh from his bones, feel the blood gush, hear his organs ripped out. *Peter Christopher*. His flesh shuddered in repulsion. The pain of being Peter Christopher forced a groan from his gut. He wanted to scream. He had to die *now*.

But they'd stop him. Unless he could get them to help him. His heart jumped. Why hadn't he thought of it before?

He rolled onto his back and cracked his eyelids. The ceiling with its map of meaninglessness spread before him, unmoved, unchanged. Martin was somewhere in the room, watching him. He lay still. The chair on the kitchen side of the dining room table creaked. Martin must be correcting assignments. Peter could still smell the hamburger and peas from dinner which Martin had eaten without him.

If he got them to help him, all the barriers would disappear. Sally could get him some kind of fast-acting painless poison. No, she'd never do it. Hippocratic oath shit. Never mind that he wasn't her patient. She was so goddammed devoted to making people well.

Martin? Martin could take him to the bridge. No, Martin had refused to help him visit Mrs. Logan. Martin would only agree to help Peter if Cohen said it was okay and they were both sure that suicide wouldn't harm Peter's health.

He felt his lips stretching into the leer he'd first felt at Mrs. Logan's. Laughter was divine, somebody wrote. It could be hellish for those damned. Those who left the world a worse place. Those for whom it would be better if they had never lived.

He flopped on his stomach and gripped the pillow. He willed himself to die. His muscles clenched. His breath stopped. With all his energy, he commanded his heart to cease its beating. It raced. Johnny's death was a ragged shard lodged in his brain. Every time he thought, it gouged deeper. He loosened his muscles. His mind immediately rushed into pain too deep for tears.

❖ ❖ ❖

Monday morning, Martin awoke with a start. He had rolled over and nearly fallen off the cot. All dark in the apartment. Cold. He'd have to check the thermostat. Last thing he needed was for Peter to come down with a cold. Peter was wheezing harshly, unevenly. Peter was hurt bad this time. Worse than the time his parents visited or Cunniption's. Maybe Martin should call Mort and ask for help. Peter hadn't spoken, hadn't eaten, hadn't moved except to thrash and shudder. He hadn't allowed Sally or Martin to bathe him or change his soggy pajamas. His face and eyes told Martin he was conscious and rational. He was in a state like none Martin had ever seen. Martin would have to call Mort. Not from the apartment. He'd walk over to Connecticut Avenue and use the pay phone. No. He didn't dare leave Peter alone.

He plugged in his shaver next to the doorless medicine chest and trimmed his beard by feel. Was he in some way responsible? Maybe he should have helped Peter find Johnny's mother. In the shower, he stood unmoving. Who was he to decide how Peter should spend the last few precious hours of his life? He dried himself and dressed. Back in the living room, he put on shoes, folded bed clothes and cot. Across the room, Peter lay on his side, his back to the room, his favorite position since yesterday. Martin gnawed his lip in frustration. No wiser than he had been yesterday, he shuffled to the kitchen. Yes, he'd call Mort.

He boiled eggs, made toast and coffee, poured juice.

"Peter, breakfast is ready."

No answer. No movement.

"You need to eat. You didn't have anything last night. You'll make yourself sicker."

Nothing.

Martin sat in the desk chair and rested his hand on Peter's shoulder. Peter quivered.

"Peter, talk to me. What happened?"

No movement. No sound.

"You saw Johnny's mother?"

Peter's body tensed.

"She wouldn't forgive you?"

A small flinch.

Martin withdrew his hand. "I want to tell you two things, Peter. One is that I love you. I want to help. Sally loves you. So does Bruce."

Nothing.

"The second is that you can't seek forgiveness from others. You have to start by forgiving the people you hold a grudge against. Maybe that means your parents. Maybe whoever it was that infected you. Last you have to forgive yourself."

Not so much as a flicker of response. Martin pulled himself to his feet. "Sally'll be here soon. I'm going to work. I'll be back this evening to relieve Sally. She's shifted to mids so that she can be here with you during the day while I'm gone. I'll be staying every night."

That afternoon in his office, Martin telephoned Mort. The answering machine gave a number where he could be reached. Martin dialed the number.

"You have a new job?" Martin asked.

"I quit my job so I can stay here. This is Billy's number."

"What're you living on?"

"Savings. The clinic helps."

"That's devotion."

"AIDS is my life now, Martin. Anyway, what's up?"

"It's Peter." Martin described Peter's catatonic state.

Long pause, then Mort said, "I've seen it before. Despair. It can be deadly."

"What can I do?"

"Love him."

Martin waited. "And?"

"See if you can get him to go and see his doctor. Get someone he's really fond of to come in and see him."

"He won't go, I'm sure. Everyone who loves him is around already."

"What about his parents?"

"Not much love lost there. Wait a minute. What about Billy? They're friends again, right?"

"Billy couldn't make the trip, Martin. He's mostly lost muscular control. Once in a while, he has brief spells of rationality and coordination, you know the Roller Coaster effect. But they're usually pretty short—an hour or two at the most."

"Rough."

"They're the hardest times for both of us. He understands what's happening. He cries. Talks about suicide." Mort swallowed. "They won't happen much longer. He's declining pretty fast. Anyway, guess you'd better count Billy out."

"Any other advice?"

"Hang in there. Your being there is more important than you realize. I don't want to be melodramatic or anything, but if Peter gets through this, it'll be because of you. And Martin . . ."

Long pause.

"Martin, you got to remember that you're Peter's *buddy*, not his keeper or boss or judge or father. It's Peter's life, not yours."

"I want to keep him alive as long as possible—"

"Huh-uh. Peter, not you, gets to decide how he'll live and die."

Martin hung up. Mort was right, wasn't he? All he'd done was remind Martin of his training as a buddy. *When it comes to life and death, let the patient make his own decisions.*

Next Martin dialed Sally. Yes, she could stay late at Peter's. He called Catherine's number. She answered.

"I want to see you," he said. "Tonight."

"I'm working."

"I'll meet you after you get off."

"I have an early class tomorrow. Maybe—"

"No maybe's. Tonight."

Catherine sighed. "Meet me at ten-fifteen at Lindy's, on I Street, between 20th and 21st."

Lindy's turned out to be a smoky, poorly lit, student hangout, half a flight of iron steps up from the street in a converted Victorian row house. The long bar, of polished but worn dark wood, ran the length of the narrow room. Martin took a booth at the back where the noise level allowed conversation and the beer smell was less overpowering.

At ten-fifteen Catherine came through the front entrance in her charcoal coat and red scarf. She spoke to several people as she made her way searching the booths. When she saw Martin, her smile cooled. Without speaking, she slipped off her coat, stuffed the scarf in its pocket, and slid into the booth. "How's Peter?"

"He's in emotional shock. What happened?"

"I told you. Mrs. Logan threw us out."

"Are you okay?"

She nodded. "I'm one tough broad."

She didn't look tough. Her dark hair had grown to her

shoulders. A curl fell over her forehead. She wore hoop earrings that made him think of her mother. In the half light he couldn't tell if she was made up. Her jeans and knitted top made her more curvaceous than he really liked.

"Want a beer?" he said.

"As opposed to what?"

"Wine?"

"I never drink wine. Too hoity-toity."

He raised his eyebrows, pursed his lips and nodded. "I see."

"Imagine. And in this light, too."

"Sounds like a personal problem to me."

"I don't allow myself the luxury of personal problems," she said. "Only universal ones."

"So your mother's disdain for beer has nothing to do with the case?"

"No more than the flowers that bloom in the spring, tra-la."

Martin lowered his head and struggled not to chuckle. He was here on an important mission.

"You're not taking this seriously," she said with a hint of a grin.

"Cut it out. I'm here to chew you out."

"Sorry." She folded her hands and cast down her eyes.

"Let's get it over with. Why did you help Peter? And hide it from me? You're smarter than that."

Catherine avoided his eyes. "Seemed like the right thing at the time. I'm sorry."

Martin shook his head. "Youth." He leaned to the side and squinted down the room. "The waiter's ignoring us."

"Wally's on tonight. Neat guy. He'll get to us as soon as he can."

"Catherine, you deceived me and fell for a line of crap from

Peter. I don't know yet how bad the damage is. Don't ever do that again. Think before you act. And don't try to fool people. You're too good for that."

An overweight kid in a white apron who looked like a refugee from day care stood by the table. "Hi, Kit." He wiped the sweat from his forehead with a stained white napkin.

"Wally, this is my dad," Catherine said.

"Hi," Martin said without smiling.

"Two drafts," Catherine said.

"How about tostados and chili dip?"

"Not tonight," Catherine said.

"We got egg rolls, too. Delish."

"Just the drafts," Martin said resisting the impulse to snap.

Wally whisked away with a flutter of dirty apron strings.

"As I was saying," Martin began.

"You're right," Catherine said. "I'm ashamed."

"Don't be ashamed," Martin said louder than he meant to. "Just . . . learn from mistakes."

"Okay. How about embarrassed?"

"Let's not play Semiotics and Semantics tonight. I'm tired."

She nodded. "Me, too. I only meant—"

Wally clunked two clear steins in front of them. "Assumed you wanted the large."

"Thanks," Catherine said, smiling up at him.

"Sure about those tostados?"

"Sure."

He scurried away.

Martin's eyes followed him. "Awful place to talk."

"Sorry."

"Stop being sorry for everything."

"I come by it honestly," she said.

"Don't be flip."

"Sorry."

"Don't be . . ." Martin stopped. "Is that a gotcha?"

She lowered her head in mock shame.

"You're not taking this seriously," he said.

"You're so much fun to fence with."

Martin tried to swallow his amusement. "Don't flatter me when I'm trying to be stern."

"I never stoop to flattery, but fun is fun."

"Catherine . . ." He took her hands in his. "So long since we've acted silly."

She nodded. "I've missed it."

He let go of her hands. "What you did with Peter was disreputable. Do you see that?"

She nodded. "Especially by contrast. When I saw you with Peter . . . I don't know. Guess I didn't know you had it in you."

"It's nothing new."

"I haven't seen anything like it in you for years. You've been playing the chump who lost out. Talk about self-centered. I stopped existing for you, about the same time you stopped fixing up the house. I couldn't even get you to play Alliterations with me."

"I had a failing marriage on my mind," he said.

"Poor excuse."

"Not an excuse. An explanation."

"Then you started treating me like a girl friend, trying to win me over against Mom."

He scanned the barroom, smarting. Kids as charming as they were naïve cavorted and shimmied to each other. They never closed their mouths. Martin could see dozens of sets of healthy, white teeth peeking through lips left ajar. The television over the lunch counter was booming, but it was drowned out by the roar of voices and laughter.

"When you left," she said, "I couldn't believe it. Betrayal in spades. High school was the saddest time in my life."

"I was wrong. I told you."

"Being with Peter has revived my dead father, the guy I had so much fun with. You really do love him, don't you?"

"Not half as much as I love you."

"He's your wayward son, isn't he, the son you never had?"

"I'm not here to talk about him."

She turned her head and gave him a sidelong glance. "Okay. Let's talk about us. If I promise to give up shameful behavior, will you lighten up?"

"Fair is fair. I'll try. I'm carrying a heavy load. Will you help me?"

"Starting tonight. Let's go dancing."

He lowered his chin and glowered.

"Remember," she said, "how we used to dance with me standing on your feet? You'd count the time and tell me about Johann Strauss, Junior, the unrecognized genius. I can dance on my own feet now."

"The last dance I learned was the bunny hop."

"And you were lousy at that."

"I'll make a fool of myself," he said.

"So?"

"You're actually serious."

"Never." She stood and grabbed his hand. "Come on. I'll introduce you to all my boyfriends at the Mad Hatter."

"We haven't paid."

"Wally'll put it on my tab."

As they clattered down the steps to the street, he realized

he'd been had. Catherine had always known how to play him like a gypsy violin.

❖ ❖ ❖

Sally's plea was pretty much the same as Martin's. Peter didn't move. Easier to face the wall than to see her in her work clothes, straight from the hospital. In the old days, before he got sick, he used to love the way Sally looked in her uniform and that pert little hat. She was about the prettiest thing he'd ever seen. He'd enjoyed making her smile, in the beginning anyway, before she got to be such a pill about his going out. Remembering, he felt tears gather in his closed eyes. First time he'd cried since Mrs. Logan. Nothing hurt more than remembering good times when the times turned bad.

Key in the door. Martin.

"Hi," Sally said.

"Go home and get some rest." Martin said.

Silence. Peter knew they were communicating with sign language behind his back. Any change? No. Did he eat. No. Did he talk? No. Frowns. The sound of cotton against wool. They were hugging. Consoling each other. Over him. What a waste.

"I'll be here by nine in the morning," Sally said.

"Make it nine-thirty if you want."

"Might as well come straight here from Walter Reed. I don't have time to go out to Potomac and change."

"Thanks for staying late and missing work," Martin said. "I'll get here early tomorrow afternoon so you can get some rest."

"Thanks."

More cotton on wool. The door opened and closed. Steps to the kitchen. Water running. Striking of a match. Gas being lit. Peter faded into sleep.

"Come on, mate," Martin said. "I fixed your favorite. Hot chocolate with whipped cream. You up to sitting at the table?"

Peter squeezed his eyes tighter.

"And an almond tart with marzipan. And French vanilla ice cream. I'll make hot fudge sauce if you want."

Why doesn't he leave me alone?

"Peter." Martin's voice was heavy as though it were about to break. "Please talk to me."

Peter didn't move.

"I know you're hurting," Martin said. "So am I."

Nothing for a minute, then the sound of the desk chair moving, straining.

"If it makes you feel any better," Martin said, "Catherine and I have cleared up some things. We had a long talk and went dancing. You scared her to death. She doesn't know why you wanted her to go with you. I don't, either. It had an odd side effect. She and I are a lot closer."

Peter ground his teeth. *You think I care about that, you silly bastard? I'm trying to die, and you tell me about getting over spats with your brat? And she's lucky. You care about her. You actually love her. I don't get it. She's nothing but the result of a moment of lust. Perverse. My father's more real than you are. He doesn't make a big deal of an orgasm while he had his cock jammed in my mother's cunt. He doesn't even like me. He wishes I weren't connected with him. He's ashamed of me. He'll be humiliated when he finds out what I died of, but he'll get over it, and his life will be easier. When he gets the news I'm dead, he'll say, "Nice goin', son. You done good."*

"Sometimes it helps if I hold you," Martin said. The bed sagged under Martin's weight. "Let me take off my shoes." Shifting, motion. "There." Martin's hand on his shoulder. "Come on, bunkie."

"Nice goin', son. You done good." That's what he'll say. What I always wanted him to say to me. What I ached to hear from him. Tears.

"Come on," Martin said. He pulled Peter's shoulder toward him, turned Peter around, leaned Peter's head against his chest, and put his arms around him. Peter couldn't hold back. Weeping cascaded out of him as though Martin had lanced his infected soul. "It's okay," Martin said. He rubbed Peter's back and stroked his hair. "It's okay."

◆ ◆ ◆

Even though Martin decided to arrange a tray with all the sweets and both a yellow and blue napkin and coffee in a demitasse, Peter ate little. He didn't say much. He told Martin he was sorry. Martin gave him a bubble bath, decked him out in clean hydrangea-blue pajamas, and put his favorite violet sheets on the bed. When Martin settled on the cot for the night and saw Peter's sleeping body at peace, he breathed easy for the first time in a day.

Peter did better at breakfast. A whole egg and juice. When Sally came through the door, Peter said hello. She went to the bed and held him.

Tired as he was, Martin taught better that day than he had all semester. He explained Mahler's use of "heartbreaking appoggiaturas" and demonstrated the use of the flatted sixth at the piano. After his eleven o'clock, he telephoned Mort.

"He broke down last night. Let me hold him. Any change in Billy?"

"He might snap out of it for a little while."

"And understand what's going on?"

"Yep."

"Ouch."

"You got to roll with the punches or quit."

"Anything I can do?" Martin said.

"Be there."

"It'll probably have to be by phone. I don't want to leave Peter alone. Guess you could say we're both living with our patients."

Mort laughed. "I don't think I'd put it that way. I'm not sure Billy would have me."

"Peter's already told me I'm not his type."

Another laugh. "Thank God we can still giggle over this nonsense we call life."

"Death doesn't make much sense, either."

"Sometimes even death is funny, Martin."

"I'm here if you need gallows giggles and grins."

"I'll call you if I come unglued."

Martin cut short his office hours and got to Peter's by four.

"Beat it," he said to Sally.

"Wow. With all this free time on my hands I might go on a jag in Georgetown."

Peter ate a respectable dinner. Afterwards, Martin searched for blankets.

"What're you doing?" Peter said.

"Paper said we're going to have a hard freeze tonight. This place isn't well insulated. I was chilly last night." He yanked a quilt and an ancient army blanket from the drawer. "Which one?"

"Quilt."

"Need a bath and bed change?"

Peter nodded.

In the tub, Peter lay with his eyes closed. Martin scrubbed.
"Want to talk about it?" Martin asked.

Peter shook his head. Martin waited. Peter shook his head
again. Martin went back to scrubbing.

Peter fell asleep early after a back rub. Martin turned down
the lights, undressed, read at the table until he was sleepy,
checked the heat, and turned in.

Settled on the cot, he felt the rough nap of the army blanket
on his cheek. Like being back in navy basic training. Sleeping
alone on a bed not big enough for him, yearning for the feel of
a woman. How long had it been? Funny. Every time the current
emergency was under control, the old aching needs came back.
What had Peter said so long ago? "If you're alone, it's because
you don't care enough to make the effort to bed a woman." It
wasn't that. He'd given up. He was old now. Mighty hard to
find any woman who'd want him. He thought of his take on the
old Groucho Marx line: "I wouldn't be seen with a woman so
hard up that she'd go out with *me.*" His mouth broke into the
beginnings of a laugh. Mort had it right. There was hope as long
as he could still laugh.

He was bone tired. His soul felt like a body after basic
training, bruised but tougher. Martin didn't know how much
more he could take. Mort was right. It gets harder and harder.
Roll with the punches or quit.

Martin dreamt. He and an eight-year-old Catherine were
roughhousing in the grass. She giggled and screamed. The sun
was low in the sky, casting long gold bars and black shadows
across the land. A phone was ringing somewhere. Martin
searched the grass and the shrubs. No phone. Of course not.
It was inside. He started toward the house. Vivien blocked his
way. The phone went on ringing. He tried to push past her. Her

earrings trembled . . .

Martin snapped awake. Another ring. He swung his feet onto the floor, felt for his slippers, edged through the dark to the desk, and switched on the light. He squinted at his watch. Two-forty.

"Hello?"

"Martin, this is Mort. Is Billy there?"

Martin laughed. "No, but Peter is. You're confused."

"I mean Billy. He's gone."

"You lost me. Gone?"

"An hour ago, he came out of it. Started talking. Crying. Said he wanted to die. Then he calmed down. Asked me to make coffee. Said he was going to the bathroom. I helped him get there, went in the kitchen. I waited and waited. Finally I looked. He wasn't there. My wallet was on the floor in the closet under my jacket. All my cash is missing. He's gone somewhere in his pajamas and bathrobe. I went all around the building. No sign of him. I'm calling his friends. I'm going to hit the streets. If he shows up there, call me, okay? Leave a message if I'm not here."

"Anything I can do?"

"I'll call you."

As Martin hung up, Peter sat up. "Who was it?"

Martin switched on the lamp by the wing chair. "Billy's gone."

Peter quivered. "He died?"

"No, he's gone. Snuck out of his apartment. Mort's trying to find him."

Peter stayed stock still. "What happened?"

Martin handed him his bathrobe. "He had one of his lucid periods. Got upset—he does that when he understands what's happening to him. Cried, talked about dying. He sent Mort to the kitchen to make coffee and disappeared."

"Jesus."

"Worst is he's in his bathrobe—in this weather."

"Talked about dying?" Peter's eyes widened. "Maybe . . ."
His shoulders quaked. "Martin, I know where he is."

"What do you mean?"

Peter's breath came in short gasps. "Oh, my God." He leapt
to his feet, lost his balance, almost fell. Martin caught him under
the arms. "Call Mort." Peter stumbled toward the desk.

"I'll call him," Martin said. "Get in bed."

"No—"

Martin took him by the shoulders and moved him onto the
bed.

"Call him," Peter said.

Martin dialed Billy's number. After four and a half rings, the
sound on the line changed. "This is Mort." A recording. "Please
leave a message after the tone." Then a ping.

"Mort, this is Martin. If you're there, please pick up." Martin
scratched behind his ear. "Mort?" Static on the line. Martin
hung up. "He's not there. Probably out hunting for Billy."

Peter thumped his feet on the floor. "Call me a cab." He
stumbled to the bureau, snatched jeans, tennis shoes, and a shirt.

"Peter, what are you doing?"

Peter threw on the clothes and yanked his overcoat from the
closet. "Goddammit, call a cab."

Martin grabbed him from behind, a hand on each arm.
"Stop it. I won't allow you to take any more risks."

Peter tried to twist free. Martin tightened his grip.

"Let go," Peter said through clenched teeth.

"Not unless you cut this out."

Peter thrashed. Martin dragged him backwards toward the

bed.

"Get your hands off me," Peter screamed.

"No."

Peter stopped fighting. He turned his head so that his face was close to Martin's. His forehead was wet, his eyes blood-shot. "You have no right to stop me from doing anything I want." He pushed his face closer. "You're a buddy. *A buddy.* Not my jailer, not my keeper, not my guard. I'll live my life as I wish, not as you wish." His spittle splattered Martin's face. His eyes, round and hard, forced Martin's head back. "And I'll die as I wish. *Now take your hands off me.*"

Martin let go. They both stumbled.

Peter buttoned his coat. "Call a cab."

"Let me go for you."

"He wouldn't listen to you." Peter tripped to the desk, picked up the receiver, and dialed.

"All right." Martin wrenched the phone from his hand. "I'll drive."

Peter was out the door. Martin flipped his overcoat from the hanger in the closet and pulled it on over his pajamas. Peter half ran, half staggered down to the hall. While they waited for the elevator, Peter folded his arms on the wall and rested his head. The doors whooshed open. Martin put his hand under Peter's elbow and helped him into the elevator.

"Straight south on Connecticut," Peter said. "Left on Calvert."

"He's in Adams-Morgan?"

"He's on the bridge."

In the car, Peter leaned back his head, closed his eyes. "Faster."

They zigzagged through the sparse traffic, changed lanes,

jumped yellow lights, ran reds. The tires squealed as they veered left on Calvert Street. In the last half block before the bridge, Martin slowed. A taxi pulled away from the curb on the north side of the bridge and accelerated past them, heading for Connecticut. They leaned forward and peered through the mud-spotted windshield.

Peter's arm whipped to the windshield. "There. On the north side."

At first Martin saw nothing. Then he made out a dark clump at the bridge rail. A man in a bathrobe lashed by the wind. He moved erratically, his feet scrabbling. His stomach was over the top bar of the railing.

"Stop," Peter said.

Martin braked.

"Kill the engine."

Billy had shifted his weight further over the railing, where he lay flailing.

"Get out quietly," Peter said. "Don't charge him."

Martin unlatched his door, pushed it open, and stepped onto the pavement. Peter was ahead of him, walking unevenly toward Billy. Martin caught up and put his arm around Peter's waist.

"Billy," Peter said in a firm voice.

Billy's movements slowed to involuntary spasms.

"Billy, it's Peter."

Billy wiggled forward and looked down. "Don't come no closer."

Peter inched forward. He detached himself from Martin and held his arm back, palm out, until Martin stopped.

"I told you a long time ago, Peter," Billy said in a drunken voice. "I told you what I'd do. I couldn't. I was too sick."

Peter stumbled to within six feet of Billy.

Billy turned his palsied head toward Peter. "We can't boogie no more, Peter. It's over, man. It's history."

Peter stepped toward him.

Billy pushed himself further over the balustrade. His shoulders were above the chasm. His body teetered, his arms and legs jerking. "Don't come no closer, Peter, or I'll let go."

Martin calculated. By the time he reached Billy, it would be too late. He forced himself to stand still.

Peter halted. His body weaved. "You got to boogie, Billy. Right up to the last. You didn't get your fair share. So you take the scraps and make them into whatever life you can. You got to boogie with whatever you got left."

"You ain't turnin' into a useless bag of shit," Billy said.

Peter lifted his hand and let it fall. "It's worse than that." He dropped to his knees, sank back until he was sitting on his heels, and bowed his head. "I got something to tell you, Billy. Listen to me, then let go afterwards, okay?"

"Won't make no difference, Peter."

"All you have to do is listen." Peter put his hands to his shoulders and leaned forward. "It was me infected Johnny Logan. I killed him."

Billy twisted toward Peter.

Peter nodded. "His mom won't forgive me."

Billy swayed forward, caught the rail, and stopped.

"I remembered what you said that night right here," Peter said. "And I realized you were right. Only with me it's worse than with you. I can't boogie anymore. I can't exist anymore. I've got to be destroyed."

"It's already happening."

Peter bent further toward the pavement. "Not fast enough.

Not bad enough."

Billy's body wobbled.

"So if you let go, Billy, I will, too."

"What're you talking about?"

Peter struggled to his feet and stumbled to the railing two feet from Billy. "If you jump, I'm going to jump, too, Billy."

Martin gasped. "Peter—"

"Stay away, Martin," Peter yelled. "You take one step, I'll go over."

Peter hoisted himself onto the top bar and lay on his belly. His face pointed downward into the black ravine while the wind ransacked his hair.

"Don't," Billy said.

"Why not? I'm so far below you in the shit bucket, you can't even see me."

"Jesus, Peter."

Peter spread his arm along the railing toward Billy. "Touch me."

Billy's husky form quailed. His arm jerked toward Peter. Their fingers locked.

"I love you, Billy," Peter said, his voice all but lost in the wind.

Billy closed his eyes and turned his face down toward the dark.

"I hurt you," Peter said. "Will you forgive me?"

"Yes," Billy said high in his voice.

"Will you forgive me for what I did to Johnny?"

"Yes."

Peter sighed, his hair flying, and eased his body forward. "Three seconds."

"Peter, don't," Billy cried.

Peter slid forward into the wind.

"Peter!"

Peter turned his face to Billy.

"Please," Billy said. "Not you."

Peter spread his arms and legs. "Three seconds." His legs rose behind him. His head tilted down toward the earth far below him.

Billy screamed. He pushed himself backwards, dropped onto the bridge, seized Peter's foot. Billy rolled into the street. Peter fell on top of him.

Martin darted to them. Billy quivered, his arms and legs out of control. Peter lay inert. Martin wrapped his arms around Peter and dragged him off Billy. Billy's voice crooned, machine-like, random. His eyes lost focus.

"Call Mort," Peter said in a broken voice.

"Lie quiet. I'll get the car."

Martin bolted to the VW and pulled it up beside the two bodies on the pavement. He went to Peter first. "Come on." He took Peter's hand and tried to pull him to his feet. He hung loose, a deadweight. Martin eased him to the ground, opened the car door, pushed forward the seat, and squatted beside him. "Put your arm over my shoulder. That's it. Up you come." He hauled Peter to the car and stuffed him into the back seat. Peter slumped sideways, his head against the window. Martin hurried back to Billy.

Billy's torso twitched like road kill. His limbs were out of alignment, his head tilted as though his neck were broken. His shoulders and hands were in meaningless, purposeless motion. His eyes rolled. Martin lugged him to the car and heaved him onto the passenger seat in the front.

From a pay phone on Connecticut Avenue, Martin

told Mort to meet them in front of Billy's building. Peter mumbled directions, straight north on Connecticut. Mort was at the curb. Together, Mort and Martin dragged Billy's undulating flesh to the elevator and into Billy's apartment.

"Got to go," Martin said. "Peter's in the car. Can you handle it from here?"

Mort nodded. "Go."

Peter was asleep, his head against the window. Martin drove up Connecticut to Quebec, parked in the apartment lot, went to the passenger side, opened the door, and pulled the seat forward.

"We're here. Can you make it?"

Peter didn't answer.

Martin put his hand on Peter's shoulder. "Come on, bunkie. We're home."

Martin shook him gently. His head lolled, then fell forward. His hair grazed Martin's face. "Come on, Peter." Martin pressed his hands on both sides of Peter's face and lifted his head. It fell back against the seat. Peter's lips were parted. Saliva oozed from the corner's of his mouth. "Oh, my God." Martin used his thumb to lift one of Peter's eyelids. The eyeball was rolled far back into the head. "Oh, my God."

Part III

Men Now

Chapter 10

Palliative Maneuvers

Peter knew his body hurt, but he couldn't feel the pain. He could only hear it baying deep in him, like a driven hound, far off, indistinct. Something hard and raw was in his throat. He tried to take it out, but a voice told him to leave it alone. He sank back into the gray brume.

A sound like distant laughter jarred him to the surface. He was in a strange room painted lurid yellow. Railings fenced both sides of his bed. A tube ran from his arm to a plastic bag on a pole. Another bag dripped liquid into him through a hole in his chest. His breathing sounded strange. The hard thing was gone from his throat. He put his hand to his mouth. A rigid plastic mask covered the lower half of his face. The air was wonderful, sweet and clear and comforting, like cold, cold water in the middle of the summer heat. He let the colorless sea roll over him.

Voices. Man in white and a nurse.

"He's awake," the man said.

Peter began his descent.

"Don't go back to sleep. That's better." The man was smiling. Cute guy. "Can you talk?"

Peter tried to say "yes," but a croak came out instead.

"Tell me your name."

Absurd. Peter wanted to tell the man so, but his voice

wouldn't cooperate. He just made mushy noises.

"Try again," the cute guy said.

"Pee . . ." Peter managed.

"What's the rest of it?"

"Turr."

"Good."

"Wh . . ." Peter took a deep breath. "Where?"

"George Washington University Medical Center. You've been here since Wednesday morning. It's Saturday. Welcome back to the land of the conscious."

Night again. Where'd the day go?.

"Let's try raising his bed," a woman said. He heard a buzzing and felt his body bending into a sitting position. "There, is that better?"

Martin was holding his hand. "Talk to me, bunkie."

"Mmm . . ." Peter began.

"Yes, go ahead."

". . arrr. Tinnnn . . ."

"That's right." Martin smiled at the nurse. "He knows me."

Peter coughed. "What hap . . ."

"Pneumocystis."

Tears filled Peter's eyes.

"You're getting better," Martin said. "Cohen is pleased with your progress."

Must remember to tell Cohen, Peter wanted to say in mockery. He couldn't. Instead, he tried another tack. "Sal?"

"She was here earlier."

"Bruce?"

"He's been here, too."

"Mom?"

"I didn't call your parents."

"Thanks," Peter slurred. He squeezed Martin's hand. "Friend . . . friend."

Pneumocystis. *Christ.*

Darkness. He awoke again. He was alone. The tube was still connected to his arm, but the line to his chest was gone. He felt his face. In place of the plastic mask was a nose piece made of rigid rubber. A small tube went into each nostril. He could take it out. Oxygen. That's what it was. He felt his chest and stomach. The skin was taut, bones protruding like sticks pressed through a deflated balloon. He felt first one arm, then the other. He'd lost more weight. How much? He slid his hand down below his waist. He was wrapped in padding. Jesus, a diaper. His stomach bucked. God, if he had to die, why couldn't it be with decency?

Something bit at his memory. He saw a blood-red scarf with Chinese characters. Above them, a face, a young face, a girl's face crumpled in weeping, the cheeks gleaming with tears, the dark hair shining.

A nurse gave him lunch—apple juice, milk shake, revolting mushroom soup, and a single saltine. His stomach began its familiar throbbing pain. He flicked his tongue over the lesion in his mouth. Larger. It stung when he drank the juice. His fingertips traced the lesions on his face. How far had they advanced?

Memory fragments flitted like scraps of distant lightning. Looking down in the cold moonlight, almost over the edge, about to fall, the wind pushing him. Somebody's fingers locked in his. *Three seconds.*

"You're awake."

Another nurse. She showed him a small paper cup holding two pills. "Can you swallow these?" He nodded. She raised his bed, gave him water with a plastic straw, and stood by while he struggled to swallow. His stomach complained.

She touched his forehead. "Where does it hurt?"

"Stomach," he stammered. "Hurts. *Hurts!*" It was getting sharper and more brilliant, this pain he had known for so long.

"It's that bad?"

His consciousness blazed with pain. His voice brayed.

She stroked his forehead. "I'll see what your doctor says."

He wished he could slide beneath the surface again. All the world was becoming pain. Flowering, billowing, red and purple, knives and razors full of pain, all biting his stomach. He was slobbering.

The pain went on and on. He couldn't stand it another minute. The minutes passed. He *had* to have relief.

A very long time later, she was back. "I'm going to roll you on your side."

He didn't care what she did.

"There," she said, "that should help." She eased him onto his back again. He tried to double up. His muscles contracted and twisted and stretched and quivered.

Slowly, the keenest edges of the pain faded. The core of his hurting got smaller, less vivid, darker. His moaning stopped. Quiet came upon him like twilight. His muscles relaxed. His body lay at peace.

Breathing deeply, he scanned the room. Night. The walls glowed. He wondered what she had done. He knew he was supposed to think about his parents, but he couldn't remember what. He wanted to immerse himself in relief and savor the dark, the wonderful silence, the tranquility in his body.

The following day, he ate solid food. His nurse appeared regularly to give him an injection. It stopped his pain and thrust him into deep restfulness. Cohen, Martin, Sally, and Bruce came and went.

Day and night replaced each other in a round robin of meals, pills, shots, and people, some in white, some in street clothes. Peter tried to take hold of time and force it to flow evenly, the way it was supposed to. He sorted through his splintered thoughts. Beneath the surface peace, he could feel his body putrefying. Would his flesh hold together long enough for him to go home?

No, that wasn't the problem. He was irritated at his inability to stick to one thought at a time. It was easier to think about his parents and even to think about dying than to remember—something. He pulled back the memory of the cold night. Cement icy under his stomach as he stared down, the wind cutting his face. A shaft of black in the air where the bridge cast a shadow. Far below him on the floor of a ravine, a road lined by leafless trees bent in the wind. A frozen creek dull beside the road. Somebody wavering on the bridge railing next to him. *Don't. Not you.* Billy. His body in constant mindless motion, tipping toward the chasm. *Three seconds.* Billy hadn't let go.

That still wasn't it. Something much scarier. He saw the dark-haired girl with the blood-red scarf. And a face with green eyes, red spiked hair. Bruce. They were in a car. Why was the girl crying? He recalled a fabric of blue print in a dark-hued room that smelled old. His book of Chinese writings. A photograph. A woman telling him to leave.

Mrs. Logan. The panic in his stomach as he had seen, unblinking, that he was unforgivable. His own grim acceptance of hopelessness. The mocking leer he'd felt on his own face. The demonic laugh. His decision. He quivered. He had done this to himself. When Johnny's mother refused to forgive him, he had willed his body to die.

Why hadn't he? Maybe he couldn't will himself to death. No, it wasn't that. He snapped his eyes open in surprise. Hope.

Poor old hope. So naïve, so foolish, so wrong-headed. Wasn't Johnny's death enough to damn him past all chance of forgiveness? Nothing would ever undo that act. Mrs. Logan would never forgive him.

Martin had forgiven him. So had Billy and Sally. They didn't count, did they? Why not? Weren't they human beings, too, like Johnny and Mrs. Logan and Peter's mom and dad? Martin and Billy and Sally did count.

He needed more. God's forgiveness—if there was a God. Forgiveness was God's job, not his or Martin's or Sally's or Billy's, or even Mrs. Logan's. So what Peter needed to do . . . He didn't know.

He sighed, his mind weary. He needed someone to help him think things through. Did he still want to die?

Who would tell his parents?

Days later—Peter couldn't tell how many—orderlies moved him from intensive care to a semi-private room. The atmosphere was more relaxed on the new floor, but his view from the window was all buildings. The bed next to the bathroom lay vacant. His nurse explained that he'd be alone unless another AIDS patient was admitted. Peter wanted to ask her how soon he would get his injection. His stomach was coming to life.

Sally breezed into the room. "Morning, Pete." She planted a kiss on his cheek. "See what I brought." She plunked a miniature Christmas tree, all tinsel and plastic, on his bed table.

He wrinkled his nose. "Lovely. Where did you find it?"

"In the gift shop. Glitzy, but I thought it might brighten

things up." She grinned. "Christmas is next Wednesday."

"I didn't know. I thought . . ."

"You've been here two weeks, Pete."

He breathed carefully. "I had no idea."

Sally looked away. "I'm going home for Christmas, by the way. Haven't seen my folks since spring. Martin will be staying at your place every night until I get back."

Peter felt a twinge of disappointment. His mind did a double-take. Martin staying at his place? Was he going home?

"I'll give Martin my parents' number." The phony grin returned. "Don't be so down. It's only a week."

Peter tried to smile. "It's morning. Why're you here?"

"Start swings tonight, so I'm free in the mornings."

"Why're you so bouncy?"

She raised her eyebrows in surprise, then shrugged. "I don't know. Guess I'm getting the Christmas spirit early."

"Is something wrong?"

"No, why?" She was smiling again. Her eyes—something about her eyes.

"Have you been crying?"

She toyed with the tree. "Nobody's had a chance to talk to you."

"Is somebody going to talk to me now?"

"Yes." She kissed him on the forehead and hurried out.

A nurse Peter had never seen appeared, drew the curtain that separated his bed from the vacant one next to him, changed his diaper, gave him a shot, and left. Something was very wrong. He couldn't think what it was. Pain killer seeped into his brain and restored quiet.

Cohen's head appeared from behind the curtain.

"What does a guy have to do to get a little nap?" Peter asked with fake annoyance. "This place has been Metro Center during the morning rush. Sal was just here."

"And now I'm here," Martin said, behind Cohen. "How're you doing?"

"Better," Peter said. "That pain medicine really helps."

Cohen pulled on latex gloves, lifted Peter's hospital gown, and pressed his fingertips into the flesh on Peter's chest.

Martin pulled up a chair next to the bed. "How do you like your new digs?"

"Okay," Peter said. "How come I got moved?"

"They needed the space in intensive," Martin answered.

"I wasn't asking you," Peter said with pretended irritation. "How come you know so much about it?"

"Doctor Cohen and I talked."

Peter looked from Martin to Cohen and back again.

Cohen removed Peter's oxygen tube. "Open your mouth." He peered deep into Peter's throat, probed, felt Peter's tongue. "Okay, close." He felt Peter's throat, put Peter's nose piece back in place, cranked the bed up to a sitting position, and drew up a chair. He had The Look.

Peter squared his shoulders.

"You can be discharged," Cohen said, "Saturday or Sunday, probably." The Look grew more intense. "We've done everything we can."

"The pneumocystis?"

"Arrested for the moment."

"Then I should improve, shouldn't I?"

"The KS has spread." Cohen absent-mindedly stripped off his gloves while he talked. "Can't control the diarrhea. You're losing weight. The pneumocystis will come back."

"How long do I have?"

"I don't know."

"Months?"

Cohen shook his head. "You could improve, but you're weak enough that I wouldn't expect it."

"Oh," Peter said.

Cohen rubbed his eyes. "So I don't see any point in your staying in the hospital. You can be more comfortable at home—with sufficient care. Martin's been in touch with the Hospice of Saint Anthony."

"Saint Anthony."

"It operates out of the Church of the Shepherd in Southeast," Cohen said. "Accepts AIDS cases. No anti-gay bias. It can provide home care until you need to be admitted, and your Medicaid will cover most of the cost. The Charbonne Clinic will help."

"And Sally and I will fill in," Martin said.

Peter shuddered. "Saint Anthony."

Martin leaned forward. "If you agree to hospice care, you're shifting from curative to palliative care. That means the hospice staff will do all it can to make you comfortable."

"So I would die . . ."

" . . . naturally," Cohen said, "with no artificial prolongation of life."

"So this is the end," Peter whispered.

The Look was acute.

Peter was trembling. "Need to think."

"Of course," Cohen said. "I'll see you in the morning." He stood. "Peter, I did my best."

Peter was afraid Cohen was going to cry. "Don't be sorry."

Cohen recovered. "See you tomorrow."

As Martin stood, Peter went rigid. "Martin, don't leave."

As soon as the door closed behind Cohen, Peter jangled like a marionette whose operator has lost his mind.

Martin grabbed him and held him hard against his chest. "Hang on."

"Tell me what to do," Peter sputtered.

"You have to decide."

"Cohen's going to let me die."

"Cohen's done all he can."

Peter's voice was failing. "I can't think what to do."

Martin tightened his hold.

Peter's body froze. "I can fight, insist that they do everything."

"That means machines."

"Machines," Peter crooned. "Science fiction at its most grotesque never dreamed of devices so horrifying. They suck your blood in and out of you, they take your breath and give it back, they drain your piss from you."

"Peter, *stop it.*"

Peter clamped his eyes shut. "Yes, I must stop that." He shook his head, gazed past Martin's shoulder. "Or I can let go and die. Without machines. Without props. Just die. With decency, as they say. With dignity." He tried to laugh. "What a crock. AIDS leaves you no dignity. I can't control my bowels. I'm terrified to see my own face. My body is rotting. You and Cohen and Sal talk about how I am to die behind my back. I have no dignity left to die with."

Martin turned his face away.

"Or . . ." Peter leaned back. "Martin, look at me."

Martin eyed him sidelong.

"I could stop my life right now. Martin—" Peter clutched is hand. "Will you help me?"

Martin pulled back.

"Bastard," Peter said without passion. "You're willing to help with the easy things. You leave me on my own for the hard ones."

"You think this is easy?"

"Why won't you help me?"

"I couldn't."

"You promised you'd stay with me at the end," Peter said. "Will you if I kill myself?"

No answer.

"Martin? Will you?"

"Yes."

"Will you try to stop me?"

Martin became very still. "No."

Peter breathed deeply, coughed once, and frowned into space. "Maybe, at the very last second, I'd think back on my life, and I'd say, what can I be proud of or pleased about, and I'd ask myself what I'd done to make up for the bad things I did. And I'd answer myself, 'Nothin'.' And then I'd die. That's damnation."

Martin moaned.

"I tried to die, Martin. After Mrs. Logan wouldn't forgive me. Now I'm afraid. I want a chance to make up for things and maybe do something good. And now I don't have any more time. What am I going to do?" Martin gawked at him. "Martin, what can I do? Mrs. Logan wouldn't forgive me."

"I don't know," Martin said.

"So I have to do it by myself."

"I can't find forgiveness for you. I can't die for you."

Peter took Martin's hand. "After I do something good, I won't mind." He raised his head and rasped for breath. "But *not now!* Not hooked up to a bunch of machines.'

"Lie down," Martin said. "You're worn out." He arranged Peter's pillows and cranked the bed down.

"Hospice of Saint Anthony," Peter said. "Why do I have to make this decision? Other people don't have to do this." His hands fondled his head.

He took a deep breath through his mouth and let it out. His eyes shut. He felt himself drifting into drugged sleep.

Martin slept poorly. The following morning, he bathed and dressed by rote and headed for the hospital.

"Morning, bunkie."

"You look like shit," Peter said with a caricature of a grin. "What're you doing for fun, there, young fellow? You gettin' any?"

"No, not gettin' any. And not having much fun. And who are you to be commenting on how *I* look?"

"Takes one to know one."

Martin pulled a chair close to the bed. "You're not making sense."

"Where is it written," Peter said with a flutter of his hand, "that I have to make sense?"

"You're feeling better. What happened?"

Peter gave him half a smile. "I told Cohen I'd go the hospice route. Now I have to face my mom and dad and tell them. *I* have to do it. Will you be here with me?"

Martin put his hand on top of Peter's. "When?"

Peter's eyes slid to the clock. "About half an hour."

"Half an—"

"I called them at seven."

"Peter, you've got balls."

Peter cocked his head. "Maybe before I die I'll be man enough to be handsome. *Je serais le plus beau.*" He glanced at the clock again. "Sometimes when you hold me I don't feel quite so terrified."

Martin encircled him with his arms. Peter pushed against him, his breath shallow. Martin could feel Peter's heartbeat slowing. When Peter's breath was calm and even, Martin said, "Can I ask you a question?"

"What if I said no?"

"When we were on the bridge, was that all an act to get Billy to back off?"

"No."

"You were really going to jump?"

"I wanted to. I couldn't stand the idea of Billy doing it."

"If he let go," Martin said, "were you going to follow—like you told him?"

"I don't know."

"That speech you made—about boogying right up to the end. Wasn't that for real?"

"Yes. *I* want to decide when to stop boogying. I don't want God or somebody elbowing me out of the way."

"What you said stopped Billy. My hat's off to you."

"I'm not sure I should have stopped him. Maybe he'd be better off dead. Besides, what right have I to change his mind? Odd thing is I convinced him but not myself."

"What *do* you want?"

"How the hell should I know?"

Martin rubbed Peter's back. "Why did you ask Catherine to go with you to see Mrs. Logan?"

"I thought Mrs. Logan would forgive me. Catherine would see it and maybe understand that she needed to forgive you. All I did was make things worse."

"No, you helped. We're closer than we've been since her mother and I separated. Why didn't you ask *me* to take you to see Mrs. Logan?"

Peter drew back and faced him squarely. "Because you wouldn't have done it."

"I would have."

"You said it was too dangerous, that it would shorten my life, that—"

"Didn't I take you to the park? Didn't I take you to that bar, even though I knew it was bad for you?"

"That was different, and you know it," Peter said.

"It was me who took you to the bridge."

"You tried to stop me. You said you wouldn't *allow* me to go."

"I was wrong. And in the end, I took you there myself. I know now that I have to let you make your own decisions. I'll try to help you to carry them out, even when I think you might get hurt."

Peter watched him. "So if I decide I want to, will you help me kill myself?"

"Martin," rasped Alicia's voice.

She stood in the doorway, one hand on her hip, the opposite shoulder thrust forward. Who was she posing for? Roger hulked behind her. Martin got to his feet.

"How good to see you," she said.

She eased into the room and her eyes darted around. First she scrutinized the empty bed closest to the door, then, with Roger at her elbow, she proceeded toward Martin. As she cleared the curtain between the two beds, she cast a glance at Peter, nodded, and returned her eyes to Martin. His stomach knotted.

Roger gaped at Peter.

Alicia's eyes flitted about the room. "Where—where's Peter? It's his room, isn't it?"

"Here, Mom."

Her eyes swung back.

Roger stumbled toward the bed, squinting. "Peter." The color drained from his face. "What happened?"

"Lesions. Caused by a kind of cancer called Kaposi's sarcoma."

"My God," Roger said.

"I'm . . ." Peter's voice cracked. "I have AIDS."

"AIDS?" Alicia said. "Who said you have AIDS?"

"The doctors."

She closed her mouth hard, swallowed, and stood very straight. "That's absurd." She began hunting through her purse. She found a cigarette and lit it. "Ridiculous. I want to talk to these so-called doctors."

"Mom," Peter said, "you can't smoke in here. Oxygen."

She dropped the cigarette on the floor and crushed it under her foot. "Now, who are these 'doctors'?"

"Mom," Peter said, "there's no question—"

"*Of course there's a question!*" she shrieked. She was pacing now, waving her arms. "How dare you even suggest . . . The whole thing is an absolute comedy. What's your doctor's name? I'll have the best men from Hopkins here this afternoon to straighten this out."

Roger's eyes quavered. "How did you get AIDS?"

Peter took a deep breath. "I'm homosexual, Dad."

Roger cringed.

Alicia stopped pacing. Her face had the aura of a deaf person, straining to hear but unable to make sense of the conversation. She weaved. Martin caught her by the arm and helped her sit.

Peter pushed the call button. "My mother's feeling faint. Could you come help her, please?"

"I don't know," Alicia said in a wavering voice, "who has told you these things. I don't believe any of this. I don't believe you would do this." She touched her fingertips to her forehead. Running mascara etched chinks in her cheeks. "I don't understand . . ."

A nurse hurried in and went to Alicia. "How're you doing?"

Alicia wept. "Not too well, dear. Do you have something you could give me to calm me a little? I've had quite a jolt."

"I'll bring you some water." The nurse went to the bathroom and returned carrying a plastic glass.

"I hoped for something stronger." Alicia drank. "Roger," she said before she had finished swallowing, "I think I need to go home. I think I need—I don't know—something—"

Roger didn't move.

"Is Peter's doctor here?" Alicia asked the nurse.

"I'll check." She scurried away.

"What's his name?" Alicia asked Martin.

"Cohen."

"Jewish?"

"I don't know."

She stood. "Roger, I think we should talk to Peter's doctor and head on home. I'm not feeling well."

Roger turned his head toward her but didn't answer.

Alicia groped at him. "I need to go home," she enunciated carefully. "I'm not up to very much."

Sally walked in.

"Sally Murdoch," Martin said, "I'd like you to meet Mr. and

Mrs. Christopher."

"Hello," Sally said. "I've heard so much about you."

Alicia swept Sally with her eyes. "You're his girlfriend."

Sally raised her eyebrows. "We were . . . very close. Actually, we still are."

Alicia grunted. "So who told him he's gay?"

Sally stammered and gave Martin a pleading look. He answered with a slight shrug.

Sally turned to Peter. "Hello, Pete." She moved to the side of the bed, put her arms around him, and kissed him.

"Don't touch him," Alicia said. "He has AIDS. Maybe he didn't tell you. He didn't tell us until just now." She snorted. "You're a nurse, aren't you? You believe this story about AIDS? How could he be a homosexual? You're his mistress. Is that what they call it now? Anyway, *you* know. How could he possibly have AIDS?" She began to pace again. "Every girl in high school was after him. What utter nonsense. AIDS, my foot." She wheeled. "Where's that doctor? I thought you said he was here."

"I don't know if he's here or not," Martin said.

"So now you don't *know* . . . Roger, come on. There's no point in staying here another minute."

Roger still didn't move.

"Take me home," she said.

Roger's shoulders sagged. "Yes, we'll go home." He turned back to Peter and studied his face, then started slowly for the door.

"No one will ever persuade *me*," Alicia said as they moved into the hall, "that Peter would *ever* have done anything like this. He's far too considerate. No, someone's gotten to him with this tale . . ." Her voice was still audible, rising and falling, gritty, grinding, but the words were unintelligible.

After her voice faded, Martin turned back to the bed. Peter was leaning back on the pillows, tilted, his arms at his side, sobbing. Sally put her arms around him.

"I told them," he whispered.

Sally held him and let him cry.

After Sally and Martin left, Peter wanted to slide off beneath the surface of consciousness. Images forced themselves on him. His mother whirling angrily at the foot of his bed, his father staring at him in curiosity and horror, Cohen and the goddammed Look. And behind them stood larger figures—Johnny, his grin in place, Mrs. Logan, Billy. Peter covered his face.

After his dinner-time shot, he wiped his eyes and blew his nose. He had to accept it. His parents had deserted him. Watching the rose and orange of the winter sunset reflected in the windows of the building across the street, he was strangely comforted. He'd told the truth to two people he loved—yes, he loved them. For once, he'd done something because it was a good thing to do.

The windows paled. Rose gave way to purple, then royal blue. Night settled like a promise of peace. Remorse for what he had done to Johnny would always be with him. And he knew he couldn't bribe God—if there was a God—by one right thing. The more he thought about Johnny, the more he knew Johnny would have forgiven him, just as Peter was ready to forgive whoever it was who had infected him. The poor bastard was probably dead now. Peter held his breath. "I forgive you."

Martin and Sally dropped by the following morning. Both were relieved to see him more tranquil. Cohen checked him over perfunctorily, an uneasy smile alternating with The Look.

"Please," Peter said, "don't look at me like that anymore."

"Like what?" Cohen asked, startled.

"Never mind."

Lunch was difficult. He struggled through split pea soup and a milk shake, grateful for his shot afterwards. The peace of the drug was descending over him when he heard footsteps.

Roger stood at the foot of the bed, avoiding Peter's eyes, fumbling with a box of candy. "They said family could visit any time."

Peter watched him move the candy from hand to hand. "Is Mom—"

Roger swallowed. "She got kind of sick yesterday."

"Booze?"

Roger nodded. "I talked to them about keeping her at home with nursing help, but they said to bring her in. Sisters of Charity." He shifted his weight. "I brought you some candy. Didn't know what you'd like. It's chocolates." He surveyed the room as though he hadn't seen it before. "Nice room. I got one at the Washington Circle Hotel, over on . . ." He pointed backwards. "I don't remember the name of the street, but it's only a block. I'll sort of stay there so I can come and see you, if that's okay."

"It's okay," Peter said.

Roger gave him a weak smile. "All right if I sit down?"

"Sure."

Roger pulled a chair to the side of the bed.

"I didn't think you'd come back," Peter said.

Roger tightened his lips and nodded.

"Didn't expect to see you again," Peter said.

"Guess not."

"I thought I might *never* see you again."

Roger clasped his hands. His throat made a grating noise. Tears dripped irregularly down his cheek to his chin and dropped into his lap.

"Peter?" he said in a strangled voice, without raising his head, "I'm sorry."

"Dad—"

"I'm sorry, I'm sorry, I'm sorry."

Chapter 11

Doin' Good

Martin marveled as he watched Peter improve. The Roller Coaster Effect. As soon as Peter got back to the apartment Sunday afternoon, he told Roger and Martin he wanted to resume brushing his teeth in the bathroom to prove he could do it. When he told his plan to Mrs. Hanks, his nurse from the hospice, she smiled sweetly, shook her head, and brought his toothbrush, toothpaste, and a basin to the bed. Once she left the room, Peter told Martin that he didn't like her at all. Martin turned away to hide his snicker.

Martin awoke Monday aware of the quiet. None of the early morning hiss and clatter of Connecticut Avenue traffic, no irritated honking from Porter Street. Christmas week. No classes, no office hours.

He peered across the room at Peter sleeping in the rented hospital bed beneath the spreading arms of an aluminum rack dangling translucent plastic bags and tubes. Martin recognized the same sense of well-being he used to feel in the first years after the divorce when Catherine stayed overnight with him. Peter was home again. But Peter wasn't Martin's child. And Cohen had said Peter wouldn't last more than a few weeks. Martin's peace persisted, undisturbed by the facts.

He wouldn't be seeing Catherine this Christmas. She'd promised her mother that she'd spend the holiday recess in

Potomac. She asked Martin not to call her there. The tension between Vivien and Martin upset her. Martin, always the odd man out in this trio, would have to wait. Again. Wait until after the beginning of the year when Catherine was back on campus.

He rose quietly, bathed, dressed, and started breakfast. While the eggs were cooking, he heard Peter moving.

Mrs. Hanks let herself in at eight o'clock.

"Morning," she breathed at the kitchen door. "He's still asleep?"

Martin looked up from the eggs. She smiled at him as she unbuttoned her coat. Her teeth were as white as the tiny pearls in her earrings, her hair frosted with silver, her eyes a warm earth-brown, and her skin was bright and sunny. A pretty woman.

"Heard him yawning a minute ago," Martin whispered.

"I don't like it," Peter said from the bed, "when people conspire about me in undertones."

"Mrs. Hanks," Martin said loudly while he prepared Peter's tray, "we are going to have to conspire in a normal tone of voice from now on. Big Ears has caught us in the act."

"He sounds cranky," she answered in the same tone. "Big Ears must feel better." She breezed into the bathroom and closed the door.

"And how are we doing this morning?" Martin asked Peter, all professional cheer. He placed Peter's tray on the bedside table and cranked up the bed.

"Fair," Peter frowned. "I'm going to ask Mrs. What's-her-name for my pain shot first."

"Her name is Hanks. Good idea. You need to eat more. I guess you'll do what you want. You're very good at being spoiled."

"Think so?" Peter said with another of his gruesome grins. "I don't need more practice?"

"You were born to it."

Peter inspected his nails. "You've got it or you don't."

"See you later, buddy. I'm off to shop before the rush. Be back by noon."

◆ ◆ ◆

After Martin left, Roger called to tell Peter that Alicia was to be released from the Sisters of Charity hospital that morning. He'd arranged for home nursing and was going to drive to Baltimore to take her home. He'd be back in Washington in the early afternoon.

A little past eleven, the phone rang again. Mrs. Hanks answered. "May I say who's calling?" She put her hand over the receiver. "You want to talk to your mother?"

Peter took the receiver.

"Hello, Mom."

"Merry Christmas, darlin'. By the way, who answered the phone?"

"A nurse from the hospice."

"You really believe that's necessary, Peter? And wise? You need to think positively."

Peter didn't know what to say. "And how are you? Dad said—"

"Might have known. You *know* how he exaggerates, Peter. Small problem quickly solved. By the way, I'm hoping you'll be able to come up for Christmas. Bud and Helen are arriving tomorrow. They're dying to see you. Ever since Robbie—"

"What?" Peter said, unable to follow her.

"They've always been very fond of you, Peter. You know

that."

"Mom, I don't think I understand." He took a deep breath. "You know I'm too sick to travel. And—I don't know how to say this, but—I'll be doing well just to make it through Christmas."

"Peter," she said, her voice rising, "I will not *allow* you to talk that way. You got to get over this depression and start thinking about getting well. Quit lollygagging around saying 'poor me' all the time. Get with it, boy. Where's your backbone?"

"Mom, when they released me from the hospital, they put me under hospice care. Do you understand what that means?"

"Never mind, Peter," she said, growing shrill. "I want you to get better. You understand me?" She broke into a raw laugh. "Why are we gettin' so serious? You need to keep things light, boy. You need to look at the bright side."

"Mom, is there any chance that you could maybe come down and see me? Maybe we could spend Christmas together. Or maybe tomorrow. Maybe you could bring Uncle Bud and Aunt Helen by . . ."

"Peter, I'd love to . . ."

"Mom . . ."

" . . . but I have a long standing commitment to Father Duncan . . ."

" . . . there's so little time . . ."

" . . . to help him with food deliveries for the poor at Christmas." She stopped and continued more quietly. "And Bud and Helen will be here."

Peter waited.

"Got to run, darlin'. Just wanted to check and see how you were doing. Merry Christmas, Peter."

Merry Fucking Christmas.

That afternoon, while Roger was helping Martin put away the groceries, Bruce called. He was getting ready to fly home for the holidays and wondered if he could stop by and see Peter on the way to the airport. He arrived at four. After Martin let him in, Bruce and Roger eyed each other. Martin introduced him to Mrs. Hanks.

Finally, Bruce turned toward the bed. Peter reached for him. Martin and Mrs. Hanks pushed aside the web of plastic tubes while Bruce hugged Peter.

"How are you?"

"Hanging on," Peter said with a husky laugh. "So good to see you. Where've you been?"

"Sick. The flu, I guess. Don't worry. I'm over it now. I'm not infectious."

"I don't think I am, either. They tell me that when you're in the advanced stages of the disease, you're not infectious anymore." He coughed. "I'd be a good date now." He glanced at Martin, Roger, and Mrs. Hanks. "Do you suppose we could have a little privacy?"

Mrs. Hanks went to the kitchen. Roger fidgeted at the dining room table. Martin returned to the wing chair and *The Washington Post.*

"They've released new findings," Bruce said in a low voice. "It was in the paper this morning. Not good news. Seems if you're seropositive there's a 30 to 40 percent chance you'll come down with it over a period of seven years."

"God. They keep increasing the odds. When did you, like, get the virus?"

"I don't know. When did you?"

"I don't know, either. Don't even know who infected me."

"I've got a 60 percent chance," Bruce said with an elfin grin. "I'll make it. I've always been good at squeaking by."

"And I've always been what they called a scrapper and survivor. Jesus, isn't that sad? Nobody's a survivor. We all die."

Bruce grimaced.

"I *am* a scrapper, though," Peter said. "When the reaper comes, he'd better come armed."

Bruce looked jarred.

"Never mind," Peter said. "He and I are on such intimate terms I just call him by his name and drop the title, the grim part. Anyway, I'm doing everything I can to hang on. I'm pushing to keep my weight up."

"What is it now?"

"A hundred and four. Been going down. I'm going to try like a son-of-a-bitch. Us terminals always need something to look forward to. We need a future. I'm looking forward to Christmas. It's only two days before Christmas, and we don't have a tree yet or wreaths or anything." He gave Martin a pleading look and raised his voice. "Martin, can we have a tree?"

"Certainly," Martin said, flustered. "There's been so much to do. I didn't get to it."

"We'll have the kind of Christmas you're supposed to have," Peter said. "We'll sing Christmas carols and lay out all the ornaments and have Christmas cakes and candy and Tom 'n Jerry's and eggnog. And we'll trim the tree." He eyed Bruce. "Wish you were going to be here."

"I don't celebrate Christmas," Bruce said.

"Wish you were going to be here all the same." Peter turned to Roger. "Hope you'll be here, Dad?"

Roger blinked and swallowed. "I will."

"Wish Mom would come."

Roger's face was emotionless. Peter nodded.

❖ ❖ ❖

That evening, after Roger and Mrs. Hanks left, Martin put on latex gloves, stripped Peter, and carried him to his bath.

"Could you call Cohen?" Peter said while Martin was washing him. "Tell him to give me something really snappy to keep me going? You know, steroids or something? I'm afraid I can't make it on my own."

"Cohen's off your case," Martin said. "The doctors at the hospice are responsible now."

"I'll talk to Mrs. What's-her-name—you know, the nurse—tomorrow."

"Mrs. Hanks? She won't be here. She's going home for the holidays. You can talk to her substitute, a Miss Struthers." Martin beamed. "I'm so pleased to see you hanging in there."

"Too much despair gives me a stomachache."

"No more despair? No more thoughts about, um, ending it?"

Peter's face clouded. "Sometimes."

"I don't get it."

Peter offered one of his ghoulish grins. "Where is it written that I have to be consistent?"

Martin scrubbed more slowly. "I have trouble following all the detours, side-steps, and cut backs in your rich inner life."

"It's hard to explain. Part of me knows that I can never be forgiven for what I did. That part wants to die. Part of me wants to boogie right through the death rattle, even though I'll look like the boogeyman. Don't be so shocked. I'm getting more explicit as I get older. Anyway, I don't think those two parts are contradictory. I don't like other people taking control. Like

Mrs. What's-her-name and brushing my teeth. One of my worst nightmares has always been being raped. *I* want to be the one who decides when and where I die. I don't want it to grab me from behind. You follow that?"

"Sort of."

"And right now I'm feeling control slip through my fingers while the rhythm of death is thumping away, getting louder and louder, deafening even. I want control back, thankyouverymuch. So I'm going to work harder at hanging on."

Martin soaked the wash cloth and held it over Peter's head. "Close your eyes." Martin tightened his grasp, and water ran gently over Peter's savaged face. "Predictability has never been one of your prominent virtues."

Peter fluttered his eyelids. "Keep 'em guessin' 'til the end and leave 'em laughin' when you go. Two of the rules of a sexually successful, dominant, dying male."

"Always heard something more like, 'Keep 'em barefoot in the summer and pregnant in the winter.'"

"Sounds effeminate to me."

Martin attempted a fake frown.

"And don't give me the 'asshole' speech again," Peter yawned. "You always end up on the losing end of that one."

"Cut it out or I'll start letting your father stay with you. Then you'd *have* to behave."

Peter's face saddened. "He wouldn't stay here. The place reeks of homosexuality. And in his world, women and paid professionals take care of the shit."

"Your illness has changed him. And—I hope you don't mind—I told him how hard it was for you to face him with the truth."

"Oh, Martin—"

"And about Billy, too."

Peter flinched, closed his eyes, and shook his head.

"So maybe—" Martin said.

"Maybe. That'd be ironic. One more indication that life is fair after all."

The next morning, Christmas Eve, at eight o'clock sharp, Peter met Miss Struthers. He liked her at first. For one thing she was pretty—trim chestnut hair pulled back from her face, delicate nose, ears like rose petals, swimming brown eyes, large sensuous mouth (Peter figured she'd give a great blow job)—and spoke slowly in a drawly, throaty voice. Breeders would probably think she was sexy. But she was too young and, Peter divined, too unsure of herself. Older nurses were so much better. She cared for Peter with a by-the-numbers methodicalness that set Peter's teeth on edge. He kept expecting her to come from the kitchen with a clipboard and a sports whistle on a cord around her neck.

As soon as she arrived, Roger left for Baltimore to check on Alicia. He was back by early afternoon. He stayed with Peter while Martin shopped for a Christmas tree.

"How's Mom?" Peter asked.

"Getting by."

"Did she say anything about coming to see me?"

"No. She asked me to stay in Baltimore until Bud and Helen leave."

"They'd understand."

"Your mother doesn't want them to know. She pretends it isn't true, Peter, even with me."

"And me. You should have heard her on the phone. You

think she's, you know, hitting on all cylinders?"

"Took me years to understand her, Peter. Among other things, she's never cared much for me. I don't think she knows what love is. She's not strong. She's always lived more in her head than out in the world. If she doesn't like the way things are, she changes them in her mind. When that doesn't work, she drinks."

"Do you love her?"

Roger pursed his lips and gazed through the window. "In a way. I was crazy about her when we were young. She was beautiful and capricious. Charmed every male on the eastern seaboard."

"You stayed with her after that was all over."

Roger shrugged. "Sometimes it's easier to bear the ills we have than to fly to others we know not of."

"I never knew you to do something because it was easy."

"If I left her I'd have to be alone—if I wanted to stay in the church."

"You used to be different. When I was little. Seemed like you were happy."

"Maybe I was. I hadn't lost hope then. Up until you were maybe six or so. After that, I buried myself in work. You have any idea how effective work is as an opiate?"

"I was never like that. I loved my work—well, dancing anyway."

"I never did. Sometimes I look back and wonder what was wrong with that kid of sixteen named Roger Christopher who thought being a lawyer was such great shakes."

"Dad, do you remember Nanki-Poo?"

"I wanted you to have a dog, not a cat."

"I think that's what made me love Nanki so much. I felt protective. You hated her, didn't you?"

"It wasn't that. I wanted you to be like—"

"Like you?"

"Like my father. He always had two or three big old hunting dogs. Quite a man. He was always out doing things, fishing and hunting and sports. I always wished he would take me with him, but he said I was too little."

"You know what I think I remember from when *I* was little?" Peter said. "It was when you gave me rides. You'd tell me to turn around, put your hands under my arms, and lift me up over your head and put me on your shoulders. You'd gallop or trot or prance and tell me you were a horse or lion or eagle."

Roger softened. "I'd ask you what you wanted me to be. Once you told me to be a dragon. You complained that I wasn't flying."

"You remember it, too."

"Such a long time ago. Makes me sad to remember."

Peter hesitated, gathering the courage for the next question. "Did you ever guess that I was gay?"

Roger bowed his head. "Maybe. I don't know. I thought of you as having settled for less than I wanted for you. I never had the guts to face up to it. I rationalized that with your breeding you'd never choose to live that way."

"I didn't choose it. I was born with it."

Disbelief flickered through Roger's eyes.

Peter smiled. "You think I'd try to fool you at this late date? You think I'd have taken up the shitty life of a gay man if I could have avoided it?"

Roger was quiet for a moment, then said, "I don't know what I think anymore."

"You're afraid it reflects on you, right? Forget it. Someday they'll find out it's brain chemistry or genes or something. Best I can tell you is that I knew I was gay by the time I was seven. Tab Hunter turned me on. Marilyn Monroe didn't."

Roger's face turned nauseous. "So you became a dancer."

"Being a dancer had nothing to do with it. I danced because I couldn't not dance."

"Could you have not slept with men?"

Peter was taken aback. "Not without living a lie."

"I didn't want you to be a dancer and a dreamer like your mother. I wanted you to be solid and reliable, a respectable man. I wanted you to marry and have children, maybe a son."

"A son." Peter's eyes went liquid. *He wanted me to have a son.* He let the breath seep from his lungs. "I was never the son you wanted. And I can't ever make it up to you."

"You're my son," Roger said. "That's enough. There's nothing to make up for. I never stopped loving you. I couldn't help seeing you and your mother as being in league against me. I'm the one who missed his chance."

Peter wiped his eyes.

"Sometimes," Roger said, "I look back on my life and I remember my mistakes and I realize I did the best I could with what I had to work with at the time. I think you did, too."

How I wish I had, Peter thought. *How I wish I had.*

That evening, after Miss Struthers left and Peter's medications and ablutions were finished, Martin arranged him in bed, hooked up his tubes, and plumped his pillows. "What do you want for Christmas Eve dinner? Chops? Steak? I bought the works."

Peter assessed the ceiling with his eyes and put his hands behind his head. "Chinese food."

"At Christmas?"

"It's very cosmopolitan to have Chinese food at Christmas, Martin." Peter sighed ostentatiously. "Let's see. Mu shih pork and a little pork fried rice, kung pao chicken and shrimp in lobster sauce." He paused. "And whatever anybody else wants."

"How about the tree?" Roger asked.

All three turned to the corner on the far side of the window. The six-foot-plus Douglas fir, already in its red enamel holder, stood tall, its outspread limbs curving upward like a high diver at the apogee of flight. A jumble of pasteboard boxes lay at its feet.

"Martin bought ornaments, too," Roger said.

Peter closed his eyes, tilted back his head, and drew in air. "You know it's Christmas when the scent of pine overwhelms the smell of rubbing alcohol, sweat, and diarrhea." He gave the tree a doubtful glance. "Maybe we could decorate it tomorrow. It's going to take a lot of energy."

Martin called the Yen Ching Palace on Connecticut Avenue and placed his order. Half an hour later, Roger and Martin moved the dining room table close to Peter's bed, set it with red paper place mats and green paper napkins, and arranged plastic sacks of soy sauce, plum sauce, and Chinese mustard in the center of a plastic wreath.

"That's really garish," Peter said.

"Knew you'd like it." Martin served Peter a small portion of each dish, ground ahead of time in the blender to make the food easier to digest. "Eat."

They listened to Bach's *Christmas Oratorio* on WGMS, all blaring trumpets and squeaky boy sopranos, while they struggled with chopsticks and egg foo young. Peter giggled when Roger dropped mu shih pork in his lap.

After dinner, Roger hugged Peter and left for the hotel. Peter drifted off to sleep while Martin cleaned up, moved the dining room table back to the alcove, and swept up bits of rice and vegetable. He went to the kitchen and washed the chopsticks.

"Martin?" said Peter's voice, still woolly with sleep. "Come here. I want to show you something."

Martin wiped his hands on a kitchen towel and walked into the living room. He snapped on the lamp on the desk and raised the bed. "What's up?"

"Not me. Haven't had it up in months. How about you? Want to mess around?"

"They never told me at the clinic that I'd get propositioned regularly. I'm going to ask them to make a note of that for when they revise the training materials."

"Spoken with all the sexual passion of George Schultz— whom, by the way, you resemble when you're testy."

"It's nice," Martin said as he wiped his hands on his towel for the third time with pained tolerance, "to see that you're feeling good enough to pass for Grendel's mother on a bad night with the light behind her."

"You're too kind. Besides that, you're stealing my material. Actually, I'm not feeling all that good. Fact of the matter is that I'm pissed. My body's not cooperating. I fell down this afternoon while I was trying to get to the bathroom to brush my teeth."

"You shouldn't have been doing that."

"I have to keep some independence, don't you understand?" Peter watched the red and green lights in the houses on Porter Street twinkle through the rain. "It's the latest in the humbling experiences this disease has graced my life with. Now I won't be able to brush my own teeth anymore."

"You're trying to take on too much. Remember, you're barely out of the hospital. Did you hurt yourself?"

Peter pointed to his forehead. "Hit my head on the desk chair. Broke the skin and bruised it."

Martin bent and studied the lump. The laceration, in the middle of a two-inch lesion, was all but invisible.

"Could have been a whole lot worse," Peter said. "Miss Struthers came apart like raw eggs in the blender. I thought for a minute she was going to spank me."

Martin suppressed a smile.

"She said that was *it*." Peter wagged his head and shook an index finger at Martin. "No more foolishness. From now on *she* was going to brush my teeth for me." He folded his arms over his chest.

"She's right, you know."

"That doesn't make me any less mad at her. I don't want her poking around in my mouth. Her brand of latex gloves smells bad. After tomorrow morning, I can tell you how they taste."

Martin sighed. "Sorry, my friend. That's the way the cookie crumbles."

"Jesus. Even George Schultz is more original than that."

"Maybe, but he's not so great at cleaning up diarrhea."

"I don't think you're taking this seriously. I really bashed myself."

"Is that anything like gay bashing?"

"Martin, that's not funny," Peter said with a forced frown.

"Sorry. I thought it was." Martin chuckled in spite of himself. "Still think so. How about some eggnog?"

Peter nodded, his face still sour. He sipped through a straw and gave Martin a scowl too theatrical to be real.

"Beautiful," Martin said. "It's so good to see you eating."

Peter sniffed. "I feel like a little kid that gets hugs for finishing his green beans."

"Takes one to know one," Martin said fatuously.

"What's that supposed to mean?"

"Haven't the foggiest. Where is it written that I have to *mean* something every time I speak?"

"Touché. You've been waiting for a chance to use that line on me, haven't you? Sometime when I was in good spirits."

"You in good spirits?"

"I feel pretty good tonight, thanks partly to you—much as I hate to admit it." Peter's face lost its animation. He bit his lip. "I want to try something. I think I'm close enough now that I can face it."

Martin placed his hand over Peter's. "What?"

"I want to see how bad I look."

"I got rid of all the mirrors."

Peter shook his head. "In the bottom drawer of my bureau."

Martin searched through the drawer until he found a round, gold-framed, two-sided make-up mirror on an art nouveau stand.

Peter leaned back, held the mirror in his lap, and covered it with his hands. His eyebrows wrinkled. "I'm scared." He reached toward Martin. "Hold me. It'll make me brave."

Martin slipped out of his shoes, sat on the bed, slid against the raised half of the mattress, and took Peter in his arms. Peter rested his back on Martin's chest and drew a long, noisy breath. He lifted the mirror in both hands and gazed into it.

In a silence so deep that Martin could hear his own breathing, Peter stared at his reflection. Slowly, he turned the mirror to the magnifying side. "My *God.*" He reversed the mirror again, lifted it above his face, and looked up into it. Finally, he pressed it against his belly. For long minutes, he lay unmoving in Martin's arms. When he spoke, he rasped so low that Martin strained to hear. "I've never seen anything like that. I didn't know such ugliness was possible." He lay on Martin's chest, breathing deeply. "Why did you let me see myself?"

He raised the mirror as if to confirm that he hadn't hallucinated. He shook his head, laid the mirror in his lap, and spread his hands over it as though to cover it from his own sight. "How can I stand to have anyone ever look at me again?"

He sat very still. Martin waited. Finally, Peter slid forward. Martin slipped from under him and stood.

"In the same drawer," Peter said, "there's a locked box. There's a gold key in the cigar box in the top drawer of the desk."

Martin brought him the box—dark wood, large enough to hold legal documents—and the key. Peter inserted the key in the lock and turned it until it clicked. The lid opened. The box was packed with letters, snapshots, an address book, and business cards. Peter withdrew a stack of glossy photographs. They were all of Peter, some in the nude, some in obscene poses. Martin tried not to notice. Peter made no attempt to hide them. He pulled out an eight-by-ten black-and-white print and handed it to Martin. It showed Peter, in the nude, standing with his weight on one leg, a sling over his shoulder. *David.*

"Destroy everything except this," Peter said. "The negative is in the box. Take it to a photo shop and have them make a blow-up from the waist up. I want to put it on the wall."

Christmas day was dark and brooding. The sullen sky echoed Peter's mood from the night before. He hadn't even told Martin good night. As soon as Martin was dressed, he spread holly sprigs on the desk and bureau and lit four squat dusty-red candles, scented with what turned out to be sugary bayberry. He decided to put the wreath—adorned with checkered sea-green-and-red ribbons and a clutch of neon-colored ball ornaments—on the inside of the apartment door, where Peter could see it. He was pounding a nail when Peter awoke.

"God, you're noisy," Peter said. "Didn't they teach you that sick people like it quiet?"

"Yes," Martin said, still pounding, "but you're a special case. Over-qualified. Besides, it's time you were awake. It's Christmas."

"What on earth is that stench? Sweet Aunt Minerva— candles? Are we having an early funeral?"

"Quit your bitching."

"Where *did* you get that obscenity you're desecrating my door with?"

"They said it would mollify postulant curmudgeons."

Peter huffed. "You, sir, are a chuffy glump."

"What's that?"

"I don't know, but doesn't the sound of it just curl your toe nails?"

Thank God Martin had his back to the room. Peter wouldn't see the easing of tension in his face. He'd been expecting the worst since the mirror episode. He switched on the radio. "The 'Festival of Carols' is supposed to be on WETA. Maybe it'll cheer you up. Merry Christmas, by the way."

Peter put his hands behind his head. "Merry Christmas to you, too, you noisy bastard. What time is it?"

"Almost eight o'clock. Miss Struthers will be here soon."

"You like her, don't you?"

"What makes you think that?"

"Something about the way you leer at her," Peter said. "You think she's sexy?"

"That's not the same thing as liking her."

"She's better than Mrs. What's-her-name."

"Mrs. Hanks?"

"Yes, her." Peter wrinkled his nose.

"Why don't you like her?"

"She won't let me go to the bathroom to brush my teeth."

"Sounds like an ego problem to me." Martin resumed his pounding.

"Fuck you."

"Is that another proposition?"

"A-ha! You're interested."

Martin forced his mouth to stay serious. "I've successfully mastered the temptation."

"Will *you* let me go to the bathroom to brush my teeth?"

"I'll bring you a basin and your brush."

"You're as bad as Mrs. What's-her-name."

"Peter, call her by her right name."

"I can never remember the names of people I don't like."

"You like her just fine. You just won't admit it. The way she frets over you. You love it, and you know it."

Peter sniffed. "If she cared anything at all about me, she'd let me do what I want."

"*I* like her. She's—I don't know—there's something about her."

"Thought as much. You're on the make for her, too."

"No, I'm not. She *is* pretty. And I *do* like her. And I'm . . . attracted to Miss Struthers."

"You men. All alike. Only after one thing."

"I'm glad your father can't hear you talking like that."

"Me, too."

They heard a key in the lock.

"That's Miss Struthers," Martin whispered. "So keep a civil tongue in your head."

"Yes, chuffy."

A little past nine Roger arrived carrying a box wrapped in white tissue and tied with K-Mart scarlet ribbon topped by a wrinkled attempt at a bow. "Merry Christmas, Peter. How are you today?" He shoved the gift on the top shelf of the closet.

"He's feeling good enough to be obnoxious," Martin said.

While Roger was hanging up his coat, Peter gave Martin the finger. Then he smiled angelically at Roger. "Merry Christmas, Dad. Did you bring me something?"

"Later. After dinner."

"By the way," Martin said, "what do you want for dinner? I told you what we have. There's turkey, too. I could put it in now—"

Peter put his hands behind his head and examined the ceiling with great interest. "Let me see. I think maybe Spanish food. No, something South American. Maybe an Ecuadorian banquet or a Peruvian feast. Something Bolivian."

"Where in the world am I going to find food like that?"

"Adams-Morgan. You can find anything there."

"Nothing's open on Christmas."

"If you care anything at all about me, you'll find south-of-the-border food for me for Christmas." Peter extended his arm and surveyed his nails. "That would make the day—what shall I call it—"

"Cosmopolitan?"

"The very word."

"On your good days, you're a pain in the ass."

"Please don't use that word in vain."

Martin opened his mouth to respond, stopped, and gave

Peter a withering look.

"You know what else might be good?" Peter said. "Sushi. Haven't had sushi in ages. Or maybe Indian keema matar with lots of curry. Or maybe—"

"Okay, okay, we'll have South American food. If I can find any." Martin grumbled wordlessly. "When do you want dinner?"

"Don't you know anything about Christmas? You always have Christmas dinner in the middle of the day."

Roger got up. "I'll be back by then."

"Where're you going?" Peter asked.

"To Mass. It's Christmas, Peter."

After Roger left, Peter said to Martin, "Would you mind letting me have a little privacy? I want to make a personal phone call."

"Mysterious this morning, aren't we?"

"Just want to wish Billy Merry Christmas. If he's up to talking. Or maybe he can listen."

"How about if I work with Miss Struthers in the kitchen?"

"Fine. No hanky-panky behind my back."

"Why? You want to watch?"

"Martin, puh-lease."

Martin put the telephone in Peter's lap and joined Miss Struthers in the kitchen. Peter dialed Billy's number.

"Hello?" said a voice. It wasn't Billy.

"This is Peter Christopher, a friend of Billy's. I'd like to wish him Merry Christmas if he's up to talking on the phone."

"Hello, Peter. This is Mort."

"Merry Christmas, Mort."

No answer.

"Can I talk to Billy?" Peter said.

"I wish you could, Peter."

"Maybe if you put the receiver to his ear—"

"Peter, Billy died the day before yesterday."

Peter closed his eyes.

"Sorry you had to find out this way," Mort said. "I'm only here to clean up. I left a message at Martin's."

"Billy died at home?"

"At the hospice of Saint Anthony."

Peter swallowed the pain in his throat. "Was he lucid at the end?'

"No. He hadn't really been in touch for a week. No pain or struggle. Just sort of faded out."

"Like he said."

"He was hoping to hear from you," Mort said. "I tried to call you last week to tell you that the end was close. I couldn't reach Martin, either."

"I was in the hospital."

"Billy loved you, Peter."

Why did Mort have to say that? "Have to hang up now," Peter said in a hoarse whisper. "Can't talk anymore."

Billy dead. He went faster than Peter, but not as fast as Johnny. Billy, who couldn't boogie anymore. Billy had lost control. *Just like me*, Peter said to himself. *Just like me.*

Martin breezed through the door to the apartment, his arms filled with brown bags, his muffler trailing behind him. "Mission accomplished. I feel like Scrooge visiting Bob Cratchit."

"You look more like the ghost of Christmas past," Peter said. "You realize how long you've been gone? A man could starve to death around here."

"Peter, cut it out," Roger said.

"Let the hell cat warble," Martin said, all grins. "If he's not good, we'll crank up both ends of his bed and let him practice being the letter U."

"You're certainly full of yourself," Peter said with unconvincing ill humor. "What did you get, a Chilean luau to go?"

"Better than that. An Ethiopian formal dinner for four."

"*Ethiopian*? That's not South American."

"It's not? Never was very good at geology."

"Geography," Peter corrected.

"Told you I wasn't any good at it. Anyway, the Eritrean in the restaurant assured me that it was *very* cosmopolitan to eat Ethiopian food on Christmas."

After dinner, Miss Struthers left for the day, and Roger did the dishes while Martin bathed Peter and changed the bed. Settled in fresh sheets and wearing his royal blue flannel pajamas, Peter asked Martin to crank up the bed to a sitting position.

"Now," Peter said, "get Dad. It's Christmas day, you know."

Martin and Roger drew up chairs, one from the desk and one from the dining room table.

Peter looked like a little boy dressed up for Halloween. "I can't wait any longer. The presents. Did anybody get me anything?"

"Don't you want to do the tree first?" Roger asked. "We've been putting it off until you were ready."

"Don't want to wait that long."

Roger rose and walked to the hall. "Never can tell what you'll find in a hall closet." He reached to the top shelf. "Why, yes, there *are* two packages here with your name on them, Peter."

He returned and put them in Peter's lap.

"To Peter from Martin Merry Christmas," Peter read aloud from the tag. He winked at Martin and tore away the silver paper and white ribbon. Inside he found a bedspread, satin to the touch and royal blue in color. "Gorgeous!"

"Not handsome?" Martin said.

"Truly handsome. Blue has balls." He embraced the bedspread. "Thank you." He picked up the other package. "'Merry Christmas Peter Love Dad.' You both need work on commas." He tore off the wrap. The paper fell away to reveal a twelve-by-eighteen color photograph in a plain frame. The picture showed five teenagers in navy uniforms, bathed in light on a stage set as the deck of a ship. Peter, boyish, dominated the group in the shining white and gold of a naval officer's uniform.

"*Mister Roberts*," Peter said. He raised his eyes. "Where did you get this?"

"Your mother had it," Roger said. "I had it blown up and framed. Thought you might like it."

Peter handed the picture to Martin. "I was a junior in high school. Got the lead." He turned back to Roger. "You never came."

Roger looked at the rug. "One of the chances I missed."

"It's a wonderful gift, Dad. Thank you."

Roger rose from his chair and embraced Peter. "Now, *now* can we trim the tree?"

"Put Christmas music on the stereo first, okay?"

When the Mormon Tabernacle Choir boomed the first note of "Joy to the World," Martin moved the yellow chair and put the fir near the window, close to the foot of Peter's bed.

"Start with the lights," Peter said. "Plug them in so that you can see what color they are while you string them on the tree.

That's the idea. Now, when you get to the ornaments, remember that the biggest ones go on first. You put one on and you stand back and hunt for an empty spot and you fill it in. Understand? Come on, everybody. On your mark, get set, decorate!"

Martin and Roger obediently trimmed the tree.

"No, no," Peter cried, exasperated. "Never put blue and gold next to each other. That suggests green, the one color you don't want. All you got was balls? Who said you have no balls? No dangles or gingerbread men or anything? Dad, there's already a red one there. Put it down lower. More to the left. No, no, no, no! Martin get that silver one away from the gold one. Ye gods. Is your taste only in your choice of women? Put that green one back in the box. Okay, now the smaller ones. Fill in where there are gaps. Not there, that's already crowded."

Martin swallowed his grin.

"Take the tinsel strand by strand," Peter said. "You want it evenly distributed. Not too close to the lights. Looks kitschy. Yeah, that's better. More on the top. Don't forget the top."

They stepped back.

"Admit it," Peter said, "it's a masterpiece, and you couldn't have done it without me."

"It's not finished," Roger said.

"What's missing?"

"The star." Roger held up a simple, old fashioned silver five-pointed star as big as the spread of his hand.

"Oh," Peter said, the bravado gone from his voice, "I didn't know we had one. It looks like the one we used to have."

"It is. Brought it from home. You want to put it on?"

"Don't think I can, Dad."

"I'll help."

Roger set the star down, walked to the bed, and pulled back

the bed clothes. "Ready?"

"What are you going to do?"

"Carry you."

Martin took the rubber nose piece from Peter's nostrils, laid it aside, removed the tubes from Peter's chest and arms, hung them over the intravenous rack. Roger put his arms under Peter's body. As he lifted Peter from the bed, Peter wrapped his arms around his father's neck. Roger carried him to the tree.

"Martin, give me the star." Peter lifted it toward the top of the tree. His sleeve fell back. His trembling white arm, blackened at the elbow and bicep with lesions, was so thin it was spectral. The fingers stretched, quavered, reached.

"Dad, move closer."

Roger took two small steps into the tree. Its branches spread and embraced the father and the son. Ornaments and lights and tinsel quivered. Both faces strained upward. Peter's shaking hand slipped the tube at the base of the star over the peak of the tree. As he withdrew his arm, they gazed up, mouths open, eyes wide.

"Now go around," Peter said, "so I can see if it's straight."

Roger edged backwards and walked slowly around the tree. Peter lifted one ball from a limb, turned it, and hung it on a lower branch. Roger moved back toward the middle of the tree. Peter turned his eyes to his father and smiled. Roger smiled, too.

"Looks good," Peter said.

"Looks good," Roger repeated. "Nice goin', son. You done good."

Peter's eyes moistened. He hugged Roger.

"Turn off the lamps, Martin," Roger said, "so we can get the full effect." He walked backwards until he reached the middle of the room.

Martin switched off all but the tree lights. In silhouette, the two figures became one, wrapped in the glow of the tree. They stood motionless and silent. Martin lifted his eyes to the top of the tree. The five-pointed multifaceted star, tarnished by time and dulled by use, caught the light and radiated quietly.

The record ended. Martin switched on the lights and took the record from the stereo. Roger carried Peter back to the bed. Martin restored the tubes to his body. Roger pulled the covers over Peter, bent, and held him in his arms.

"Crank the bed down, will you, Dad?" Peter said. "I'm so tired." He stretched. "A friend of mine died two days ago. Just found out. It was Billy, Martin. I wondered which of us would be first." He reached for Martin's hand. "Martin, the Ethiopian food was better than a Christmas goose. Truly cosmopolitan. Now, I have New Year's to look forward to."

Peter closed his eyes. His breathing slowed. Roger tip-toed to the kitchen. Martin could hear him finishing the dishes. Martin collected the tissue, foil, and wrinkled red and white ribbons, put the ornament boxes in the closet, arranged the new bedspread over Peter, and set the *Mister Roberts* picture on the desk where Peter would see it when he woke.

The kitchen light went off. Roger went to the closet, put on his coat, and came close to Martin. "Good night," he whispered. "Merry Christmas." He let himself out and closed the door silently behind him.

Billy was dead. Peter was fighting to hang on. Martin made up the cot and changed to pajamas in the bathroom. The last thing he saw before he fell asleep was the tree. It still shimmered, topped with a glowing silver star.

Chapter 12

Snow

Three days until New Year's. Martin's eyes moved to the pictures above the bed—Mister Roberts, undaunted innocence and nobility in shining white; and David in all his sensual glory, eyes bright and alert, the sling held ready over one perfect shoulder. Martin looked back to the shrunken creature in the bed. Peter had lost his brittle forward drive. He still talked about New Year's, but the conviction was feeble. His eyes had taken on a rheumy glaze Martin had never seen before. His movements had developed a fast jitter like an old movie. Sometimes, especially when he was awakening from one of his long naps, he didn't know where he was. Could this wasted body, blackened with lesions, ninety pounds of stretched skin over jutting bones, could this body last three days?

After breakfast, Mrs. Hanks signaled Martin to meet her out in the hall.

"You're back early," Martin said.

"I wanted to be with him when he dies."

"How did you know? He was in better shape when you left." She shrugged. "I knew."

"How long?"

"Days."

"Weeks?"

"Days," she repeated, her brown eyes sharp. "He's losing

ground fast. Don't know what's keeping him alive. His body is destroyed."

"The KS?"

"He's failing on every front."

"Maybe he'll bounce back," Martin said. "He's done it before. The Roller Coaster effect. And he's still eating."

"He hasn't got much left to keep alive."

"What can we do?"

"Love him."

Same answer Mort gave him. He wanted something concrete. He wanted to *do* something, He was going to protest, but her face stopped him. Defeated, he nodded and started in.

She caught him by the arm. "It's time to take him to the hospice."

Martin's throat ached. "How long can we hold off?"

"Two, three days."

"I'll talk to him. You're sure?"

Martin searched her eyes. She nodded.

Every day since Christmas, as Martin watched, Roger had stayed by his son. When Peter slept, Roger grieved, dry-eyed, anguished. When Peter woke, Roger's face glowed with caring.

"Dad, you look terrible," Peter said Tuesday morning. He slurred his speech like a drunk. His eyes were glazed.

"I probably should be getting more rest," Roger said.

Peter shifted his body. "It's New Year's Eve. I'm going to make it to 1986." He waved toward the wall. "I'd like Martin to have the picture of me—the David. It's not in my will. You can take Mister Roberts—if you want it. And the new bedspread." He rolled his head toward Roger. "Would you say good-bye to Aunt Helen and Uncle Bud for me?" His face turned sad. "Tell

Mom I forgive her and ask her to forgive me."

Roger nodded.

"Will you tell her that I love her, too?" Peter said.

Almost at once he was asleep.

Mid-afternoon, Peter's fever began to climb. Mrs. Hanks examined him, her face sober. She woke him for medicine and liquids. "Got to keep the liquids flowing, Peter. It's very important."

He drank through a clear plastic straw and scanned around the room as if it were strange to him.

Late in the day, Martin went to Adams-Morgan and bought serpentine, confetti, paper hats, balloons, a bottle of sparkling cider, and a three-foot high rooster piñata, a picaresque parody of an overwrought bird, rendered in screaming red, yellow, and orange, and sporting real feathers, dyed purple and green. When he returned to the apartment, he sidled in and deposited his packages in the corner of the dining alcove where Peter was least likely to see them before New Year's.

Peter slept motionless in coma-like calm. Still in his coat, Martin stood over him fretting. When Mrs. Hanks slid her hand into Martin's, he questioned her with his eyes. She gave him a sad smile.

Peter stirred. She fed him water, then telephoned the hospice and asked to have nurses attend Peter around the clock until he checked in. When she left for the day, another nurse, who introduced herself as Peggy, relieved her.

Before dinner, Martin put on latex gloves, spread towels under Peter, and washed his body with a cloth dipped in warm scented bubble bath. Satisfied that every trace of sweat, urine, and diarrhea was sponged away, Martin patted him dry with a soft towel.

"Feels good, huh, bunkie?"

Peter shrugged. "Nothing feels good anymore."

"It's time to move to the hospice, Peter."

Peter's eyes opened wide. "It's that close, huh?" He shivered. "My mind never failed did it, Martin?"

"You were lucky."

"I don't want to go. It's like a hospital, isn't it?"

"Pretty much. A lot calmer and quieter, though."

Peter shivered. "You've got me scared again. Do they have machines there?"

"You already signed the living will."

"I still don't want to go."

"You can stay here, but we can't make you as comfortable as you'd be in the hospice. They have the staff and equipment to—"

Peter stopped him with a wave. "Tell you what. Admit me to the hospice on Thursday. Let me spend New Year's here."

"Deal."

The morning of New Year's day, Peter didn't waken for breakfast. While Martin stood behind her, breakfast tray in hand, Mrs. Hanks stroked Peter's head until his eyelids fluttered. "Liquids, Peter." She slid the clear plastic straw between his lips. "Come on, you can do it." The lips closed around the straw. Juice rose reluctantly toward his mouth. When the plastic cup was half empty, Peter's lips separated. Two streams of orange ran down his chin. Mrs. Hanks set the cup aside and wiped his face. "Good work. That's enough for now."

She straightened, glanced at the tray in Martin's hands, and gave her head a fast shake. Martin took Peter's breakfast back to the kitchen.

When Roger arrived, he spelled Mrs. Hanks, waking Peter

every hour to drink. Close to noon, Martin squatted in the corner of the dining alcove and opened his packages. He stored the cider in the refrigerator and stashed four stemmed glasses in the freezing compartment. In strict silence, he and Roger inflated the balloons, tied them in clusters, and taped them to strings hung from the ceiling. Serpentine, confetti, and hats went on the coffee table. Martin propped the rooster piñata on the desk chair beside the bed.

At noon, Mrs. Hanks took Peter's hand. "Lunch time, Peter."
Peter groaned.

"I'm going to crank the bed up," Roger said.

As the bed came up, Peter rolled his head back and forth and cracked his eyelids. "No rest for the wicked," he said indistinctly. "The wages of sin are . . ." His eyes blinked open and focused on the piñata. " . . . a great big cock." He squinted. "With feathers." The corners of his mouth turned up. "Did I die and go to heaven?"

"Happy 1986," Martin said. "You made it."

"New goal," Peter said. "Twelfth Night."

"January sixth?"

"Think I'll make it?" Peter's eyes caught the bunches of balloons hanging from the ceiling. "Looks like someone got sick in here. Call the orderly."

"We didn't want to wake you up at midnight," Martin said, "so we put off the celebration until now. Champagne with lunch?"

"Me?" Peter snorted. "The shape I'm in? What're you sniffing?"

"It's really cider."

"The bubbles will clog my straw. And what's with the *coq aux plumes*?"

"A piñata. You want to break it open? You can use the broom handle."

"Right after my morning jog."

"It's tied to a stick. I could hold it up—"

Mrs. Hanks gave Martin a disapproving frown and fast head shake. "How about some lunch?"

Peter gave her a frown. "Were you and Dad in on this apartment-polluting binge?"

"Strictly Martin's doing," Roger said.

Peter nodded. "Got his fingerprints all over it. *Gaucherie tout flamme.*"

"Watch out who you call a faggot," Martin said. "I know French, too, you know."

Peter scanned the room. "I don't know about you, Martin. Your aesthetic sensibilities are suspect. And likely to remain that way. Good God. Serpentine, too?"

Martin flushed. "Sorry. Thought you'd want to celebrate."

Peter extended a shaking hand. "Nice job, bunkie. You're a sweetheart. And the best buddy a dying queer could hope for."

Martin took his hand.

After Mrs. Hanks forced as much food as she could into Peter, he asked to have the bed cranked down and slipped into sleep. Martin and Roger took down the balloons and hid the New Year's paraphernalia under the dining room table. When Peggy arrived, Roger said goodnight to Peter and shuffled to the door.

Peter ate little dinner and said nothing. He was more at peace than Martin had ever seen him. After the dishes were washed, Martin sponged Peter's body and put dry pajamas on him. Peggy brought his evening ration of pills and capsules and gave him an injection. Martin turned off most of the lights in the room and changed into pajamas in the bathroom. Peggy checked Peter, arranged her night light on the dining room table, went into the bathroom, and closed the door. Before settling himself on the cot, Martin glanced at Peter. He was awake.

"Martin?"

Martin walked to the bed.

"Thanks for the balloons and piñata," Peter said. "Scrumptious."

Martin blushed. "Guess they weren't very appropriate."

"That's what made them so hilarious."

"You didn't laugh."

"Laughing hurts. I avoid it. They cracked me up, though. Perfect for a Peter Christopher New Year's."

Martin eased into the chair. "Thanks for telling me. I was pretty embarrassed."

"One more thing. When am I supposed to go to the hospice?"

"We set it up for tomorrow morning, remember?"

"Oh." Peter lay silent for a moment, then said, "I don't want to go, Martin." He scanned the black winter sky through the window. "This might be the time I talked about."

"The time . . ." Martin began.

Peter rolled his head back and locked his eyes on Martin's. ". . . when I kill myself."

Martin froze.

"Will you help me?" Peter whispered.

Martin pulled air into his lungs and fought off an impulse to flinch. "Yes."

Peter stared past Martin's shoulder. "I told my parents the truth about me. I have one thing to look back on at the last minute. Only one good thing out of a whole lifetime. Not much, is it?"

"That's not all. Thanks to you, Catherine and I are back together."

Peter's lips parted. "Really? I did that?"

"Yeah. It worked in a way you didn't expect."

"Jesus. I screwed up, but I get credit anyway."

"You did what you set out to do. I owe you."

Peter smirked. "Slipped that one over on God."

"You saved Billy, too."

"That was a good thing?"

"You risked your life for him."

Peter chortled, coughed. "That's like gambling with stage money."

"You did it. You gave up some of what little life you had left for Billy. If you hadn't gone to him that night, you wouldn't be so sick now."

"Lot of good it did," Peter said.

"You did the best you could."

"Not much to bribe God with, is it?"

"It's enough."

"You really think so?"

Martin nodded.

Peter looked past Martin again. Martin waited.

"No," Peter said. "I don't need . . . Killing myself now would be inefficient." He gave Martin a fair approximation of a wry smile. "I'll let it ride. It won't be long, anyway." He closed his eyes and let his body relax. The serenity returned. "I'll go to the hospice."

Martin sat on the edge of the bed and put his hand over Peter's. "Are you so frightened?"

"Stay with me while I get settled. I won't be scared

anymore." He tipped his head toward the David and Mister
Roberts above him on the wall. "Will you hang them over the
bed at the hospice? I want people to see me the way I used to be.
And bring my new blue bedspread."

◆ ◆ ◆

The room, one of only eight at the Hospice of Saint
Anthony, was bright with early morning sunshine from the
wall of glass behind the bed. Martin checked everything one
last time. He stood back and surveyed, trying to see as Peter
would see. The walls were canary yellow, the sheets a sky blue.
The chrome of the hospital bed, the ash-colored steel of the
racks holding acetate bags and tubes, and the harsh metal of the
oxygen cylinders paled under the glow of the dozens of yellow
roses Bruce had sent. Their heady fragrance filled the room,
hiding the hint of bleach and isopropyl alcohol in the air. The
photograph of Peter as David hung on the wall to the left of the
bed, Mister Roberts to the right. Martin turned back the covers.
The new bedspread showed, even with the sheets and blankets
folded over it. Good.

The door swung open. Roger propped it with a rubber
wedge. "Hope we didn't keep you waiting. Traffic." He wheeled
Peter in. "I drove like an old woman."

Martin squatted by the wheelchair. "What do you think,
bunkie?"

"Nice," Peter said. "No check in or anything."

"Martin took care of all that," Roger said. "Let's get you into
bed."

"It's pretty." Peter glanced around as Martin lifted him into
the bed. "I have my pictures and my bed spread and roses. From
Bruce?"

Martin nodded.

"It isn't so scary after all."

"I knew you'd like it," a familiar voice said. Mrs. Hanks. "I'll be your nurse during the day. If you need anything, use the call button."

"I thought you were assigned to outpatient work," Martin said.

"I asked to be on days here so I could go on taking care of Peter." Her expression told him the rest.

Martin, Mrs. Hanks, and Roger worked as a team. In minutes they had Peter ensconced in bed and hooked to his tubes and oxygen, a phone within reach, and his call button pinned to his pillow.

"Now," Mrs. Hanks said, "what can I get you?"

"Do you suppose," Peter said, exuding creaky charm, "that I might have a piping hot cup of fresh, black coffee?"

"Right away." She bustled off.

The muscles in Peter's face loosened. "Almost done." He put his hand over Martin's. "You suppose Billy died in this room? Or Johnny? Or maybe even the man who infected me? Maybe they did. It's a nice room. I hope they did." He let go of Martin's hand. "So tired. Time to rest." His eyes fluttered closed.

"I'll stay with him," Roger whispered. "And drink the coffee. Take some time off, Martin. Good behavior."

Martin drove back to the apartment. After taking down the Christmas tree, he put on gloves, stripped the bed, and gathered Peter's diarrhea-stained pajamas, towels, and wash cloths into the laundry. While he was vacuuming, he moved the dining room table into the middle of the alcove. On the floor against the wall he found the piñata, bags of confetti, shriveled balloons. He lifted the piñata by its stick and turned it slowly. Pretty garish.

Peter was right. The embarrassment came back. Silly thing for
Martin to do. What the hell was he going to do with all this
stuff? He tore open a cellophane bag of serpentine, fished out a
pale lavender roll, and fingered it. Holding the end against his
palm with his thumb, he heaved. A curling stream of lavender
cut across the room like sleepy lightening. With a sigh he knew
nobody could hear, he gathered the used paper streamer into the
garbage.

When the dishes were finished and the kitchen and
bathroom cleaned and sterilized, he called the rental company
to come for the bed, oxygen, the racks, tubes, and bed table. He
called Mort and left a message on his machine. "Thought I'd call
and see how you're holding up. By the way, you have any use for
some confetti? And a piñata in the shape of a cock? I mean, not
a *cock*, but, you know, like a rooster? Colorful. Feathers and all."
He hung up and blushed. Why the hell did he say that? Peter's
joke. Not very funny. Not very tasteful. The words had stuck in
his mind. Freudian slip? *Why can't you erase messages on someone
else's answering machine? Or even in our own head?*

He checked the refrigerator. Loads of food. He opened the
freezing compartment. Steaks, chops, the turkey he'd gotten
for Christmas. Maybe Mort or the clinic could use some of
it. He started to dial Mort's number again and stopped. God
only knew what he might say this time. He dropped into the
desk chair. All those hours, days, and weeks with Peter had
changed him. He'd said words, been places, done things he never
would have believed he'd had in him. He'd given up biases and
stereotypes. He'd gained insights. He'd learned about living from
a dying man. And he had to watch his language when he was
around breeders.

Back in the kitchen, he moved the step stool in front of the sink and climbed high enough to reach the top cabinet. When he opened the door, dust powdered his face. Ought to get a rag and clean. Like pottery warriors in a Chinese tomb, the Scotch and gin stood sleeping side by side. He took the Scotch bottle by the neck and felt the rough grain of grime on glass. He stepped down, wiped off the bottle, opened it, chunked ice into a tumbler, and poured a finger of Scotch. The tart aroma bit his nostrils. No gagging. No moist palms.

He walked to the living room and settled in the wing chair, held the glass above him, and swirled it. The ice clinked, the amber liquor danced. He deliberately sniffed the Scotch. No nausea. No twinges in the brain. He sipped. The trickle burning its way down his throat grabbed his attention. He'd forgotten how fierce straight Scotch was.

Back in the kitchen, he dumped his glass in the sink. He could drink Scotch without thinking about death. Maybe it was because everything else around him these days reminded him of death. Made him want to live, made him savor the feeling of blood pulsing in his body, even made him enjoy his own unrelieved, nagging horniness. He filled his lungs, relishing the silken flow of air past lips and teeth and tongue, through his throat into his chest. Quiet and free, unclogged, unhampered.

Not for Peter. The familiar hurt clutched his heart. Peter tried so hard. He hung on no matter what. Why didn't he let go? Didn't he know we all lose in the end? Instead, he kept finding things to look forward to. What did he have to look forward to now? Twelfth Night, for Christ's sake.

What did Martin have to look forward to? What would life be like after Peter?

As the January sun settled toward the horizon, Martin drove back to the hospice. When he went to the desk to ask if he could see Peter, the willowy, blond young man (gay?) told him that buddies could come and go twenty-four hours day and gave him a key to the side entrance.

Roger sat by Peter's bed, his face a mask of strain. The bed was down, Peter's eyes closed.

"How about a break?" Martin whispered. "I'll take over for a while."

"What?" Roger blinked.

"Go for a walk or something."

Roger took his overcoat from the closet, wrapped himself in it, and plodded out. Martin sat.

Peter's eyes flickered. "Martin?"

"Yep."

Peter's hands twitched. "Raise me up."

Martin cranked the bed and poured ice water. "Here."

"Spare me. Mrs. Hanks and Dad are pumping so much fluid into me I feel like I'm all bladder."

"Drink."

"If you care anything at all about me, you'll let me stay dry."

"Drink."

Peter appraised him. "Guess my charm isn't all it once was."

"You going to drink or do I have to get the enema bag?"

Peter managed an exaggerated frown and took the straw between his lips. He drank half a glass. "You guys are creating an economically unhealthy bull market in the diaper trade."

Martin allowed himself a small grin. "Feeling better?"

"They changed my medication. I stay stoned."

"It's more than that." Martin played with his beard. "You've been different since you came home from the hospital."

"Yeah. The gnawing in my belly stopped."

Martin's grin slipped. He furrowed his brows.

"I sort of came to terms with a lot of stuff," Peter said.

"Johnny?"

Peter gave him a shaky nod.

"Mrs. Logan didn't forgive you," Martin said.

"One of the things still hurting me is thinking about her—all bitterness and venom. She isn't like that. I did that to her. What a fool I was to go and see her. I had fantasies of how it would be, all 1950's movie stuff. She straightened me out real fast. I hurt her."

"I don't understand," Martin said. "I thought you wanted her forgiveness more than anything."

"I forgave myself. While I was still in the hospital, I understood for the first time. Forgiveness is God's business. Not ours. The best we can do is let go, and then God can forgive us. I don't know. Maybe there is a God. Maybe he forgave me."

"You know something, young man? You're awesome."

Peter's mouth formed a close-lipped smile. "I know."

"Seriously." Martin avoided his eyes. "You've taught me so much."

Peter smirked. "Most of it was bullshit. I lie a lot."

"Thanks anyway."

Peter's smile faded. "I learned from you, too, about decency and caring enough to do something really well. The sad part was that you never let me help you."

"You did help me, in a way you never knew. Remember the day you sent me away? Catherine didn't want to see me anymore. I thought my life was over. Then you called me."

Peter studied him. "I think I knew that somehow." He lay silent. "Have I done everything now, Martin? Can I let go?"

"What about Twelfth Night?"

Peter waved it away. "Oh, that. Seriously. What do you

think?"

"You have to decide."

"Bastard," Peter said. "You always do the easy things and leave the hard ones for me to handle by myself."

"I'll be here. But you have to do it. I can't do it for you."

"What about Dad?"

"You don't need his permission."

"Sometimes he sits by the bed watching me. Makes me so sad. Sometimes I feel like I should hang on for his sake."

"Why don't you ask him?"

Friday morning, after Martin left for the apartment to do laundry, Peter slept. Late in the morning, he forced his eyelids to flutter when he felt a hand on his shoulder.

"Dad?" Peter said.

"It's me."

"Need to tell you something. Don't know how to say it."

"Say it," Roger said.

Peter opened his arms. Roger leaned forward and held him.

"I love you, Dad," Peter said. Peter felt him nod. Peter snuggled closer. "A person doesn't check into a hospice expecting to check out again." Roger nodded again. "Wanted to be sure you knew." Peter tightened his grip on Roger. "I'll always grieve that I didn't live up to your dreams. I was one of those poor spirits living in gray twilight. I tried to do better when it was too late."

Roger pulled back. "Too late?"

Peter steeled himself for what was coming next.

Roger clapped Peter on the shoulder. "Don't you know how proud I am to be Peter Christopher's father?"

Peter stretched his eyes open. Roger's face was wrinkled into a smile, large and broad, showing white, perfectly shaped teeth like Peter's had been once. Roger's midnight blue eyes were moist.

"What about Robbie?" Peter said. "He dared mighty things—"

"So did you, my son. So did you."

◆ ◆ ◆

Late in the day, Martin buttonholed Mrs. Hanks in the hall. "He won't last much longer," he said.

"I don't know. He's sparking along today. You think it's Twelfth Night?"

"I think it's the medication. He talked about letting go. I promised him I'd be with him at the end. Will you call me if you think he's going?"

"I'll give you a beeper. Whoever is on duty will page you when it's time."

That night, Martin telephoned Catherine. She was due back from Christmas recess. The girlish voice on the other end of the line told Martin that, yes, Catherine was back, but, no, she wasn't in right then. Martin left a message.

By Saturday, Peter had stopped eating. He fell into deep sleeps. When he was awake, he was polite but distracted, as if listening to other voices. His speech became more slurred and monosyllabic. Slowly, his eyes lost their focus.

When Martin came to the hospice Sunday morning, Mrs. Hanks told him that the room adjoining Peter's had been vacated and Roger was moving in.

Peter was awake but gazed vacantly, as if hypnotized. Martin took the chair next to Peter's bed and spoke to him. Peter answered with incoherent noises. Not knowing what else to do, Martin waited by the bed in silence. Finally, he took Peter's hand in his own and held it.

Peter's eyes focused. "Mar'n."

"Yes, bunkie, it's me."

"Mar'n." Peter turned his head away as if someone had spoken to him. He squeezed his eyes shut, reopened them, and looked in Martin's direction. "You know what?" He sounded stoned. "You know what?"

"What?"

"We're not . . ." Peter shook his head sharply and emptied his body of air. "We're not no-accounts anymore," he said with effort, carefully pronouncing each syllable. "We're men now."

"That's right."

"You, too," Peter said. He sighed once. "Got t'go now. Robbie." He closed his eyes. Martin put his ear near Peter's nose. Peter was still breathing.

That night when Martin got home, he found a scrawled note taped to his bedroom door. "Sally called. She's back. Call her." She answered on the first ring.

"He's pretty far gone," he told her. "He isn't aware of what's going on around him a lot of the time. I guess we got him to the hospice just in time."

"Or maybe he was waiting until now to let go," Sally said. "I've seen a lot of that. People have more control than we think. I'll stop by tomorrow night."

"Okay. I'll plan to be gone before you get there. They try to keep the number of visitors down. Otherwise it turns into Dupont Circle at Friday rush hour. I don't know if Peter will know the difference, but, Sally, if he's conscious, tell him it's January sixth. Tell him it's Twelfth Night. Tell him he made it again."

At home early the next night, Martin found himself with nothing to do for the first time in months. January sixth. Twelfth Night. He doubted that Peter knew or cared. What next? Valentine's?

After dinner, Gary, Craig, and Stan trooped to the basement to watch Monday Night Football on Craig's booming big-screen television. Martin washed dishes. He didn't need to be with them. He could hear every detail of the game through the vibrating floor.

The sink was filthy. He scoured and bleached it and started in on the counters. The cabinets cried out for attention. So did the window over the sink. And the stove turned his stomach. The refrigerator smelled of decomposing vegetables and putrid meat. The linoleum was the color of grime-ground-into-grease. Almost before he knew it, he was into a full-fledged cleaning frenzy. He ignored the questioning glances and disapproving remarks during Stan's periodic trips to the kitchen for beer. Between television commercials, Martin heard Gary say, "Martin's, like, an okay dude, you know? Just a little funny. Age does that to you. Shit, let him, like, scrub all he wants. Whatever." Laughter.

At midnight, Martin gave up. He hadn't even touched the walls or oil-caked ceiling, and the stove was only half-done. He showered and searched for pajamas. They were all at Peter's. Besides, since when had he worn anything to bed at home?

He slid between the sheets feeling that he'd forgotten something. The bed felt alien. The room was a stranger's. He didn't belong here anymore.

Martin tried to call Catherine Tuesday night and again Wednesday morning. She didn't return his calls. Were the young voices on the other end of the line vague and evasive, or was he imagining things?

Wednesday night Peter slept through Martin's visit. Martin drove home from the hospice in a stupor. His mind kept engaging in nonsense dialogue about Catherine mixed in crazy sequence with visions of Peter's empty eyes, focused on nothing. Why didn't Peter die and leave them all in peace? Why was he dragging it out?

Martin jumped. What the hell was he thinking? Wishing Peter dead? He emptied his lungs and gave his head a sharp shake. He'd learned during training that those closest to the dying person sometimes had inadvertent thoughts like this. Knowing it was one thing. Doing it was something else.

He let himself into the house. No stereos with strident cries, no booming voices or raw laughter. He was closing the door when she spoke.

"Hello, Martin."

He spun. Vivien perched in the chair near the piano.

She wore large gold hoop earrings, like the ones she wore the night she threw him out. Her dress was a fashionable tan wool, and her sunny hair was swept up from her neck to the top of her head where it lay in lazy curls. She was smiling through lips that seemed naturally colored. Her long, narrow hazel eyes, made narrower by her smile, glinted with rootless graciousness. Her skin glowed warm, pink and tan, healthy. Her body, relaxed and confident, challenged him.

As his surprise passed, Martin was awed again by her beauty. Even in her forties, she was the most beautiful woman he had ever seen. He knew that she was wearing make-up—she always did—and he knew that the effect she created was completely deliberate. He knew that she was being provocative when she crossed her legs that way, so properly that he couldn't fault her for it. The result was a small electric shock in men like Martin. He *knew* it was all calculated. She still left him breathless.

"Hello," he said. "How did you get in?"

"Your house mates. They were all headed for Frisbee's, whatever that is."

Martin watched her, his lips parted. "You all right?"

"Fine."

"Would you like coffee?"

She shook her head, and her hair rippled as if breezes were playing through it. "I wouldn't turn down an offer of a drink."

"I don't have much. There's probably beer."

She wrinkled her nose. "I've never cared for beer. You know that."

"I have some not-very-good wine."

"Maybe a glass of white."

"All I have is red."

"Fine."

He hurried to his room, stripped off his top coat, and threw it on the bed. He found his jug of wine, carried it to the kitchen, and poured. She sat, waiting by the piano. He handed her a stemmed glass.

"None for you?" she asked.

"Not now."

She was playing him. It made him wary. Why was she trying to charm him? Habit? He wavered under her spell.

She sipped. "You were out late."

"I've been to visit my patient."

"Oh," she said with a solicitous twang, "the man with AIDS.

Catherine told me. How is he?"

"Dying."

"I'm sorry." She sipped, her eyes on his. "I haven't seen you in such a long time, Martin. You're looking well."

"I'm not, but thanks for the thought."

"What's going on in your life these days?"

"Teaching. Taking care of Peter, my patient. Seeing Catherine sometimes. How about you?"

She laughed. "I'm getting married again, Martin."

"I didn't know. Who—"

"Arnie."

"Your boss?"

"He's more like my partner these days."

"Thought he was married."

"Divorced years ago."

Martin fidgeted. "May I ask you a personal question? Do you love him, Vivien?"

"That *is* personal. Let's say we're comfortable together. Arnie and I have known each other for years. You know that. We've both been alone for some time, he longer than I. We've comforted each other. We're compatible." She cocked her head. "I think we're a good match."

Martin wanted to ask her how long Arnie had been fucking her. Since before she and Martin had split up?

"Martin," she said, "are you *jealous?*"

He turned away. "No."

"I think you are."

"You and I were married a long time. It's not easy to think of you with another man."

"Don't you think you're being slightly sanctimonious, considering your record?"

"I never loved anyone but you."

"You showed it in a most peculiar way. You humiliated me in front of everyone. You and—what was her name?—Hedda."

He squeezed his eyes shut and clenched his teeth.

"I'm sorry," he heard her say. He opened his eyes.

She was looking at the floor, her eyes rumpled like tired silk, her hands knotted. "I don't want to quarrel. I need your help. Catherine's been seeing a divorced man. She stays weekends with him. I told her I wouldn't stand for it. She stormed out of the house and said she'd never come back. She even threatened to move away. She never returns my calls."

Martin frowned. "She can't have known him long. At Thanksgiving, she had no place to go."

"She met him at some party or other in early December."

"She hasn't had much time to spend with him."

"You wouldn't understand. You've never been particularly concerned with sexual mores. She barely knows the man. And she spent the weekend with him."

"You mean, she spent *one* weekend with him?"

"Martin, she's only eighteen. It's . . ." Vivien twisted. "It's *shabby*."

"That's what you fought about?"

"That's not all. She's also brazen enough to object, yes, actually *object*, to my marriage plans. She had the gall to tell me that if I married Arnie she'd never speak to me again. I mean, how dare she pass judgment on me, *me*, when she, herself—"

Martin shook his head. "I have the feeling that there's more to this story than you've told me. Which did you fight about first, Arnie or this man she's seeing?"

Vivien re-crossed her legs. "Actually, Arnie got involved. He stayed over at the house on Christmas Eve. I told him about this man she was seeing, and he . . . counseled her. And she blew up."

"Jesus, Vivien—"

"Please don't swear."

Martin closed his eyes and nodded. "Why are you telling me all this?"

"Maybe she'll listen to you." She daubed at her eyes. "Talk to her. Tell her—"

"That you're sorry?"

"I'm *not* sorry. She had no business—"

"What should I tell her?"

Vivien started to cry. "I don't know. I don't want to lose her." She gave way to weeping, her face in her hands, all pretense gone. "I love her, Martin. More than I realized. I want her back."

He listened to her voice rise and break on the sobs. He knew her voice so well. He used to love that voice. Now, he tried to deflect her pain, but he couldn't.

"Okay," he said. "I'll talk to her." He scratched behind both ears. "I'll tell her you love her."

"Thank you," she said, her face still in her hands.

He watched her weep. He wanted to comfort her, but he didn't want to touch her. Her sobs subsided.

"Would you like more wine?" he asked.

"No." She sat up and wiped her face, careful to avoid smearing her make-up. "I have to be on my way. Arnie's parked outside."

Martin glowered out the window into the night. He could see nothing. He hadn't noticed any other cars when he parked.

She got to her feet. "May I use your bathroom?"

"In the hall."

When she returned, her self-assurance, her poise, her perfect grooming were all in place again.

"Sorry I carried on so, Martin." She hustled around the room. "Now, where did I leave my coat?" She found it, a blue, full cashmere, draped over the piano bench. She put it on, adjusted the cowl collar, and checked to be sure that the gold circle pin was straight. She picked up her purse from the chair and put her handkerchief in it. "Call me and let me know, will you?" The tone was elegant and impersonal, but her eyes, for a moment, pleaded with him. She took his hands in hers and brushed her lips across his cheek. Now she was smiling again, at ease and confident. She went out into the night and closed the door behind her without a sound.

Martin stood looking after her. He heard a car door open and close. An engine started up. Headlights swept the window.

Her smell lingered—a faint scent of wools and cashmere, a tinge of musky perfume, a hint of wine. Beneath it all was the aroma of Vivien herself, cinnamon and summer sunshine.

Martin fell into the chair she had occupied. It was over. His unquenchable desire for her had died. Arnie could have her. Martin would be content. And yet . . .

Something of himself had died. His youth, perhaps? He shook his head. He didn't hate her anymore. He didn't crave her, either. She was one more human being with strengths and flaws and nobility and compulsions like all the rest. He could help her, now that his life no longer depended on hers.

Why did growing up take so long and hurt so much? Why did Peter have to know he was dying before he could live? Why did Catherine have to go through such suffering to come to terms with her parents? Was there a better way?

Why did he, Martin, have to wait until now, when the yesterdays outnumbered the tomorrows, before he could take on life free of major distortions? He sighed. Count your blessings.

Vivien still hadn't grown up. Maybe she never would. At least Martin had time left in which to live. Why do we all have to be so terribly, terrifyingly human?

And Catherine? Now he understood why she hadn't returned his calls. She was raging again. He couldn't blame her. Vivien and Arnie. He shuddered. He reached for the telephone.

"Hello?" answered a sleepy voice.

"Catherine?" He heard a scrape as she adjusted the receiver.

"You know what time it is?" she said.

He checked at his watch. After midnight. "You all right? I've been trying to reach you."

"I didn't want to talk to anyone. I needed time to think."

"Your mother told me about the—what shall I call it?—disagreement you two had."

"Disagreement?" She laughed. "It was a brawl. Did she tell you about Arnie?"

"They're getting married."

"About time. They've been sleeping together for—I don't know when they started."

"I guessed as much," Martin said. "When did you find out?"

"Christmas Day. When I got up, Arnie was still there. That was their way of letting me know what was going on. Mom got furious with me. Arnie gave me a talking to. Made me sick. I told Mom I couldn't see that what I did was any different from what she was doing. That's when she hit me."

"My God. Catherine, I'm sorry."

"*Don't be sorry!* You're always sorry."

"This time I should be." He scratched behind his ear. "I want to see you. When can we get together?"

"I don't know. I'm trying to think through things. I want to see you before . . . Daddy, I'm going to leave Washington and go somewhere else. I need to be on my own."

Her words hit him like a sledgehammer to the gut.

"You remember that scholarship at MIT?" she said. "I called them and told them I could be there for the spring semester."

Martin swallowed. "When're you leaving?"

"Friday night. The semester starts Monday. I've told GW. I can get part of my tuition and board back for Mom."

"Does she know?"

"Haven't told her."

"She'll foam at the mouth, Catherine."

"Now I don't have to depend on her anymore. The scholarship will pay for my tuition and lab fees, and they said I could get a job."

"What will your major be?"

"Double major, math and computer science."

"I thought you wanted to study something in the hard sciences, chemistry or physics."

"I can't get a scholarship in science. I have to get away."

He sighed. "I hope you're doing the right thing. It's so sudden. Just when we were getting to know each other."

"I have to do it."

"What about the man you're seeing?"

"I wasn't *seeing* him. Didn't really like him much. He was crazy about me—in a selfish sort of way. Will you take me to the airport Friday night? I know it's a bad time, but I had to take the cheapest flight."

Martin chewed his lower lip. "I can't. I promised Peter I'd be with him at the end. He could die any time."

"I want to see you."

"Maybe tomorrow if he's better."

"Can't, Daddy. Got to finish packing and clear out the room

and talk to the university administration people and borrow money and . . ." She paused. "How about Friday afternoon, before I leave?"

"Okay. Can you meet me at the Hyatt Regency? It's only ten minutes from the hospice. You could get a limousine from there."

"Better than that, I can get Allen to pick me up there."

"Allen?"

"I told you about him. He lives near our old house in Potomac. Anyway, he's going to GW, and he said he wanted to take me to the airport if you couldn't. Why don't you meet me at the Hyatt an hour before I have to leave for the airport?"

"I'm sorry about this," Martin said. "I promised Peter. What time?"

"Four-thirty okay?"

"Fine." His chest was hurting. "I don't know what I'm going to do with you so far away." He stopped himself and closed his throat. "I love you, Catherine."

"I love you, too, Daddy."

❖ ❖ ❖

When Martin arrived at the hospice Thursday morning, Roger was trying to feed Peter.

"Come on, son," Roger said. "you've got to eat."

Peter's eyes wandered uncomprehending. What was left of his face looked permanently surprised.

"Sally came by again last night," Roger said. "She's a pip. I don't think he knew who she was. She took it in stride. Come on, son. One bite." Roger put a spoonful of something that resembled mush between Peter's teeth. "He won't chew or swallow." Mush dripped from the corner of Peter's mouth.

"Don't try anymore," Martin said. "He doesn't want to eat."

Roger sighed. He wiped Peter's face and cranked the bed down. As he did, Peter swallowed. "There," Roger said with a smile.

"You must be exhausted." Martin put his hand on Roger's shoulder. "Why don't you sleep for a little while? I'll call you if anything happens."

"Don't leave him alone," Roger said, his eyes wide. He rose, rolled the hospital table away from the bed, and lumbered through the door to the adjoining room.

Martin sat by the bed. He took Peter's hand in his and rubbed it. "Hello, Peter. It's me, Martin." Peter continued to stare off into space. "How're you doing, bunkie? You were right. I didn't let you help me. Will you help me now? I want to tell you something. You have to listen, that's all." Martin sat back, his hand still on Peter's. "Catherine's going away. She needs to be on her own, away from her mother and me. I think she's wise to do it. It hurts, Peter. I don't know what I'll do without her."

He took a tissue from the box beside the bed.

"Why do I always lose people just when I find them? Catherine will be gone. I've only had you since last summer, and now I'm going to lose you, too. What am I going to do?"

He bent forward and rested his forehead on the bed next to their hands. Peter's hand withdrew in small jerks and went over Martin's. Martin raised his head. Peter had not changed position. His eyes were closed.

"Peter?" Martin said.

Peter made no response. His breathing was shallow.

From the hospice, Martin drove to the Lincoln campus. Time to get materials ready. Classes started Monday. He scanned his harmony class notes. First session. Intervals and the functions of the seven triads native to each key. Pitfalls of the tritone and parallel fifths. Avoid doubling the third. Late in the day, he helped a young woman rearrange her schedule, drop a course in piano, and add one in choral conducting. He was doing everything he was supposed to do.

No phone calls. No beeper pages. To be sure, he telephoned the hospice. Mrs. Hanks reassured him. Nothing had changed.

He walked to the snack bar in the Student Union. As he stood in line to pay for his coffee, he heard snatches of conversation.

"So, she said she wanted to do it up in one of those Madonna looks," a girl was telling her friend. "I *told* her she'd look awful."

"Or lime," a man was saying. "Grass can't grow if the soil is too acid. Not now. In the spring."

Martin walked away from the counter past the small tables.

"He's a method actor, anyway," a young man was saying to the girl sitting with him. "The man has no soul."

" . . . when they went against Dallas last year," someone was saying.

" . . . a new transmission. You have any idea how much they want for that?"

" . . . or I might cut class. Like I care."

"Maybe we could get together tonight."

" . . . yeah, if it doesn't snow."

What were these people thinking of? Didn't they know life is so short it's terrifying? Was anything in their lives important? Did they love anyone?

Friday morning Martin reviewed his notes for Music of the Romantic Period. He'd start by playing his students a little Mozart and a little Beethoven. See the difference, he'd ask. Yes,

Mozart was in a way a precursor of the Romantics, he'd agree, especially in his last works. The *Requiem*, for instance.

He left the campus a little after two with his mind on autopilot and drove by reflex. He saw what was happening. He was shutting down, numbing himself, as if to buffer incoming shock waves. He'd activated the opiate. Too many bad things all at once.

At the hospice, Roger bent over the bed holding an arrow-shaped gray-green synthetic sponge attached to a popsicle stick. He pressed the sponge against Peter's lips until Peter opened his mouth. "That's it, son," Roger said. When he pushed the sponge between Peter's teeth, Peter closed his lips around the stick and flexed his cheek muscles.

Roger glanced over his shoulder. "He's stopped drinking. Got to keep pumping in the liquids." He pulled the sponge from Peter's mouth and dunked it in a glass of water on the bedside table. "It's mint flavored, Mrs. Hanks said. As long as he keeps sucking liquid, he's not too close." He rubbed Peter's lips with the sponge. Peter opened his mouth. "By the time he's through with it," Roger said, "it's almost dry."

"How about I relieve you?" Martin said. He let the sponge soak for a moment and slid it into Peter's mouth. Peter sucked, like a baby. He seemed unconscious although his eyes were open.

At four-fifteen, Martin checked his watch.

"I'm going to see my daughter off," he said to Roger. "She's moving to Boston. I should be back in an hour or so."

By four-thirty he was at the glowing glass entrance to the Hyatt. The crush of Friday afternoon traffic turning up New Jersey Avenue from D Street suffocated him. He raised his head to the pewter sky and inhaled the carbon-dusted air. The clouds shifted. Looked like snow.

"Hello, Daddy."

Catherine stood before him in an olive-drab raincoat, black muffler and gloves, and a knitted forest-green beret.

"Catherine." He put his arms around her and held her against him. Her muscles shifted as she stood on tip-toe to kiss his cheek. He felt her warmth. He was back on the Potomac lawn in the failing light of a fall day, sipping coffee, his child in his lap.

"It's so good to see you," she said into his ear.

They stepped apart. He put his hands on her shoulders. "You look like a student."

"I am one."

"That's a switch. You used to dress . . . I don't know . . ."

"Like a yuppie. I'm poor now."

He reached for his wallet. "Let me give you money."

"Not yet. Let me make it on my own for a while."

"Let me know. Give me your address."

"I don't have any place to live yet."

"Call me as soon as you're settled. Collect. You can always stay with me if you need a place. It's cold up there. Did you pack lots of warm clothes? Do you need a place to store stuff?"

She gave him an affectionate poke. "As usual, you're a little late with the offers."

He winced.

"Never mind. Just scratch behind your ear, and I'll know you're really flummoxed."

He looked at the sidewalk behind her. "No luggage?"

"It's in Allen's car." She gave the sky a worried glimpse. "Want to walk?"

They linked arms and wandered down New Jersey Avenue toward the mall.

"How're you doing?" he asked as they crossed D Street.

"Excited. Really on my own for the first time. I talked to Mom, by the way. She foamed at the mouth, all right."

He walked on for a moment in silence. Finally, he said, "Catherine, I hope you'll make up with your mother. She cares about you."

She grunted.

"Maybe she hasn't always," he said.

"She has Arnie."

"You're her only child. Forgive her, too, Catherine."

"No promises," Catherine said.

"I won't give up. Not for her sake. For yours."

They walked to the mall and turned toward the Capitol.

"So pretty here in the summer," she said, "when the fountains are going and all."

"It's pretty now. Just different."

"So gray."

"Gray isn't ugly."

She looked at the sky. "Wish it would snow. So graceful when it snows."

They walked through the parking lot, past the reflecting pool and monumental fountain, across the street, through the gate to the capitol grounds, past the spot where the mammoth tree had stood at Christmas.

"Did you get down to see the decorations this year?" he asked.

"No. Did you?"

"No."

They climbed the steps of the Capitol, still arm in arm. Pearl-colored flakes were dropping.

"It's snowing," he said.

"I got my wish."

"First snow this year."

At the top of the steps they turned and viewed the mall in the gathering darkness. Snow was coming down steadily.

She pushed closer to him. "Think it will stick?"

"I hope so."

Lights came on one by one in office buildings along the mall. In the distance, the Washington Monument emerged like a shining resurrection against the failing sky. Street lamps flickered, as if uncertain of themselves. Snow spiraled down, blue in the beam of the arc lights along the mall, butter-yellow in the glow of the Victorian street lamps at the edge of the sloping lawn. The Capitol behind them sprang into light in an unheard whoosh.

"I didn't know they lit it in the winter," she said.

"The law knoweth neither time nor season."

"Shakespeare?"

"James. Martin James. I made it up. Just now, as a matter of fact." He couldn't see her face. He put his arm around her.

"Magnificent, isn't it?" she said. "Guess I'm going to miss it after all."

"I'm going to miss you."

"Me, too, Daddy."

"We were getting to understand each other. As adults, I mean."

"I liked that," she said.

"I thought you hated it."

"I did, but I liked it, too."

He looked at his watch. "What time is Allen meeting you?"

"Five-thirty."

"We'd better start back."

It was snowing hard now. They could hear the flakes and smell them and feel them.

"It's sticking, Daddy."

"I got my wish, too."

In front of the Hyatt, a red sports car waited, its engine running. Martin took her in his arms and held her.

"Write me," he said. He didn't want to let her go.

She made no move to leave his arms. "I love you, Daddy."

"I love you, Catherine."

She kissed his beard. He let her go. She hurried to the red sports car and got in. It pulled away into the falling shimmer of flakes. Martin waved. He couldn't tell if she had seen him. He watched until the car disappeared, swallowed in the blur of snow.

Martin drove to the hospice. Falling through the beams of his headlights, the snowflakes were stationary. It was he who was moving, upward on a slant, into the winter night. The illusion made him dizzy, but he preferred it to his own thoughts.

As he walked down the hall toward Peter's room, Mrs. Hanks came toward him, her face tense.

"Martin, wait."

"What is it?" Martin said, abruptly angry for no reason.

"Peter just died."

Chapter 13

Ashes

Martin blinked.

"I wanted to catch you before you went in," Mrs. Hanks said.

"When?"

"Just now. I was going to page you—"

Martin went numb. He leaned against the wall. "His father—"

"We were both with Peter when he died."

Martin's body clenched. "How's Roger doing?"

"He's holding up fine so far."

Martin's mind jolted. So much to do. "Do me a favor? Call Sally Murdoch and Bruce Dushinsky right away?"

"Will Mr. Christopher be making the funeral arrangements?"

"Peter wanted me to handle it. Is there any hurry?"

"We should remove the body as soon as possible."

Martin stood paralyzed, trying to decide what to do first. Realization shot through his brain. "I promised to be with him at the end."

She put her hand on his arm.

"I let him down," Martin said. "I failed him. I was out walking on the mall. I promised him. *I promised.*"

"I'm so sorry, Martin," she said. She put her arms around

him.

Martin pulled back. "Don't."

He went into Peter's room. Roger was by the bed, holding Peter's hand. Two vases of flowers, pink carnations and yellow roses—one each from Sally and Bruce—rested on the table under the David photograph. Martin put his hand on Roger's shoulder.

"We lost him," Roger said in a voice with no depth.

Martin squeezed his shoulder.

"He was having a terrible time with Mrs. Hanks," Roger said. "He held the sponge in his mouth and didn't suck on it. He quit, as if to say, 'Screw you. Enough's enough.'" Roger smiled at Martin, his eyes pierced with grief, and turned to Peter. "No one will ever know how much I loved him. He's my son."

Roger caught his breath and frowned. "God. I have to tell Alicia." He scowled at the room as if trying to get his bearings. "I have to go home. She's not strong. She'll need help." He struggled to his feet. "Tell Mrs. Hanks I'll be back for my things." Martin rose and accompanied him to the door.

Alone, Martin sat by the bed and took Peter's hand. "Goodbye, my friend," he said aloud. "As God is my witness, I loved you, bunkie. I don't know what I'm going to do without you." He gripped Peter's hand. "I let you down. I promised to be here with you at the end, but you didn't cooperate. You died so suddenly—"

Pain erupted in his belly. He got to his feet and fought for control.

Peter's body lay on its back, half covered by the blue bedspread, the pajama top unbuttoned. Martin had thought that nothing could ever destroy the exquisite shape of Peter's head. Death, in its own resolute way, had the final word. Peter's head was shriveled and misshapen. His eyes were half open, the rotting skin of his face contorted in a gaping grin. His arms, chest, and neck reminded Martin of a cartoon stick figure. Hair still shadowed his chest to the base of his neck. His hands were far too large for the rest, his fingers outstretched as though he had been reaching out at the moment of death. Grotesque. A revolting caricature of a former god done in poor taste.

The hair on the back of Martin's neck rose. Without Peter's spirit, the body was discarded garbage, best disposed of quickly. He slammed his eyes shut and reopened them to drink in the picture of Peter's torso on the wall. He shifted to the picture of the lad in white and gold. Peter had been a glory to look at, even then. But neither the beautiful nude nor the innocent lad was Peter any more than the repulsive cadaver in the bed. In those days, Peter had kept his spirit poor, dormant, drugged in the pursuits of narcissism. Only toward the end had his spirit been free. Only in dying had Peter been man enough to be handsome.

Martin yearned to weep. He turned away from the body, stood motionless. His heart was pounding. He felt sweat dripping down his back. He had to . . . something.

First, he sat next to Peter's body and called the funeral director recommended by the clinic—one willing to handle AIDS cases. Next he carted the roses and chrysanthemums to the front desk, to be donated to another patient. Mister Roberts and David came down from the walls and into a box along with the bedspread and Peter's spare pajamas and bathrobe. He put on gloves and swept all the items Peter had used—plastic water pitcher, cups, straws, the popsicle stick—into a black plastic garbage bag. He wanted to strip the bed, but the body still lay there. He stood in the middle of the room, arms apart, legs bent, ready to take on the next task. *What else, what else?*

He wouldn't allow himself to look at Peter. He knew as if by instinct that one glance would freeze him into inaction. He needed to keep going, to keep doing. His eyes flew around the room.

As he stood braced for action, he heard high heels in the hall. Mrs. Hanks came to the door, her coat buttoned, a muffler at her throat, one gloved hand holding the other glove.

"Martin," she said, "the staff can take care of all this. Come on. Let's get a bite to eat and—"

"I want to stay until the funeral director takes the body."

"No need. We have people—"

"I don't want him left alone."

She took a step toward him, hesitated, turned, put on the other glove, and walked out of sight.

He closed the door and went back to the bed, careful not to let his eyes rest on Peter's body. He collapsed into the chair, buried his face in his hands, and waited.

At eight-thirty, the door opened. A slight, balding man with a thin beard, dressed in a business suit and quiet tie, stepped into the room. "I'm Abel Springer, Springer Funeral Home."

Martin introduced himself.

"You might want to wait outside," Springer said.

Martin nodded and withdrew to the visitor's lounge with its orange plastic furniture, weary magazines, coffee pot, and fluorescent lights.

By nine o'clock, Peter's body was gone and arrangements for the cremation completed and paid for. Martin returned to the room and stripped the bed. Where should he take the dirty laundry? He left it in a heap in the middle of the mattress. He checked to be sure he had all of Peter's things in the box, ran his eyes around the room one last time, and turned to leave. He stopped, dropped into the chair, picked up the telephone, and dialed Mort's number.

"Mort, Peter died."

"Oh, Martin . . ." Mort was silent for a moment, then continued in a rush. "I'm so sorry. How are you holding up? Is there anything I can do?"

"Nothing I can think of." Sweat was soaking through Martin's shirt again. He loosened his tie for the third time. "Listen, Peter wanted his disease and death kept quiet for his mother's sake. I'd appreciate it if you'd ask the clinic not to mention him in any of its public stuff—you know, newsletters or announcements or anything."

"Of course. Martin, are you okay?"

"Yes, there is something you can do. Does the clinic have anyone who can help me with Peter's tax return?"

"Call Manny Hughes. He's our legal and tax advisor."

Martin was speaking faster. "By the way, Peter left some of his furniture and a little cash to the clinic. When the will's probated, you'll be getting it. In the meantime, I'm going to have to clean out his apartment. Can I ship the furniture to the clinic or somewhere?"

"No problem. Call me Monday at the clinic."

Martin's mind raced. *What else, what else?*

"Martin," Mort said, "don't push so hard."

"So much to be done all at once."

Mort grunted. "Have dinner with me next week? How about Wednesday at six-thirty? At a little place called Annie's on 17th Street."

Martin hung up. Tomorrow, he'd have to face tasks he couldn't do in the middle of the night. He had to go home, get some rest.

The following afternoon, as "the designated and only custodian" named in Peter's notarized letter about the disposal of his body, Martin picked up Peter's ashes from the funeral director. They were in a pale, pinkish-tan wooden box barely a foot square. He took them home.

Sunday Martin went to the apartment and began the long process of collecting and packing Peter's belongings. No one lived here now.

In his aching aloneness, Martin wanted to see Catherine. He couldn't call her—she didn't have a phone yet. So he stumbled through the days numb. Mornings were the worst. He'd waken slowly, move about his daily routine, and get ready to go to the apartment, then with a small stab of terrible surprise, he'd remember. Peter was dead. He died Friday afternoon. At the hospice. The words rang empty in his mind. They made no sense. They neither hurt nor comforted him. He pushed his thoughts aside, blanked them out. In off-moments, he was haunted by the specter of Peter's wasted body lying hideous in the hospice bed, arms outspread, dead eyes staring through half-closed lids.

On Wednesday night, after missing several turns, he finally found Annie's Steak House on 17th Street Northwest. He paused before the plate glass wall at the front and peered in. A dozen tables were arranged in the carpeted oblong. At the right rear, he could make out the end of a bar extending back into the darkness. He searched the tables for Mort. A face caught his eye. Big guy, blond, wool shirt open so far down he looked undressed. Jeans too tight. Martin struggled to place him. In a dark bar. Peter weeping. *Joey.* Peter's friend—his courtier—that Martin had met at Cunniption's. Maybe Martin should tell

Joey Peter was dead. Walk up to the table and say, "Excuse me. You probably don't remember me, but I was Peter Christopher's buddy. Anyway, I thought I'd tell you he died Friday. Have a good evening." No way.

Inside, he found Mort waiting for him at a table toward the back along the wall across from the bar.

"Quieter back here," Mort said.

Martin ordered a Bombay martini. He didn't know what to say. He made small talk. He thought of asking about Billy's death, decided against it. He avoided Mort's eyes.

"You haven't mentioned Peter at all," Mort said over the entrée and their second round of drinks. "You've talked about classes, your daughter, reports about the rumored new wonder drug AZT, and your roommates. What about Peter?"

Martin felt a rush of anger. "What do you want me to say?"

"Tell me about him."

"His body was horrible." Martin began, surprised at himself. "I wasn't prepared by the training or anything in my life to deal with that."

"Why was it so horrible?"

Martin talked about Peter's missing essence, that spark which made all the difference. When Peter was alive, how he looked didn't matter. When he was dead, it was the only thing that mattered. Such a lesson in the inconstancy of the flesh. Peter had been beautiful, no question about it. No, gorgeous but not handsome.

And Peter's parents, the rift between Peter and them, Peter's courage in breaking the news to them, the faithfulness of Roger, the withdrawal of Alicia. Peter's rescue of Billy. Peter's reaction to his ravaged face in the mirror. Sally and Bruce, Christmas, Thanksgiving, the visit to the bar on P Street, the trip to the park, the fight over lasagne. What was he was going to do to fill his days now that Peter was gone? When would he grieve?

Mort sipped his coffee. "You're doing it now."

The restaurant tables were all empty. The oblong was dark. A handful of men still clustered at the bar lost in a haze of cigarette smoke. Dessert had come and gone, as had an after-dinner drink and coffee, another drink, more coffee.

"Go on," Mort said.

Martin breathed hard. "Haven't told you the worst. Peter wanted me to be with him when he died. I promised. He died without me. I failed him at the most important time. I keep thinking about that."

"That must hurt."

Hurt? Yes, it hurt. He could still see Peter, stepping into the bathtub, asking Martin if he had a beautiful cock. He could hear Peter's voice demanding South American food. He could see Peter's face, stretched with grief at Cunniption's. He saw him lying in bed, extending his arm and examining his nails. The vision of Peter's face, twisted with fear, rose before him. Peter, asking Martin to hold him. Peter, saying how scared he was. Peter, pleading with Martin to be with him at the moment of death. The opiate was dispelled. Martin's pain tore through the surface of his consciousness like shrapnel. He was breaking down in public. He didn't try to stop. Nothing mattered except that Peter was dead. Martin had let him down at the final moment. He held his head in his hands and wept. Mort reached across the table and grasped his shoulder.

Finally Martin wiped his face with his napkin. "I'm so sorry. Didn't mean to embarrass you."

"You didn't."

Spare conversations still sputtered along at the bar. Martin glanced over his shoulder. No one was watching them.

"You did a magnificent job, Martin," Mort said as he walked Martin to his car. "It's people like you that make me proud to be in this business. Peter's life—and his death—would have been utterly different without you. Let's get together in a week or so. Give me a call and we'll find the time for a few laughs."

Martin chortled in spite of himself. "Like we did tonight?"

"Don't know when I've giggled so much."

"You're weird."

"Occupational hazard. Hang in there, brother."

He tapped Martin on the bicep with his fist and walked up 17th Street into the darkness.

Martin arranged for Peter's memorial service to be held in the tiny high-vaulted Chapel of Saint Theresa, just off the vestibule of the Victorian-Gothic Church of the Shepherd, whose poor and mostly black congregation sponsored the Hospice of Saint Anthony and, unlike most of its counterparts, welcomed gays. The tattered basilica, in Southeast Washington, had seen its salad days in the early nineteen hundreds. The Chapel of Saint Theresa, maybe once a baptistry, was all brown and dusty cream wood, lit by a single peaked window of frosted glass high enough in the wall that no one trapped in the room could escape. Before the other mourners arrived, Martin placed Peter's ashes—the case looked for all the world like an oversized cigar box—on a card table in the middle of the chapel's floor, a mosaic of inch-wide gray octagonal tiles. The table and its human remains lay directly beneath the frown of the larger-than-life painted wooden statue of Saint Theresa who stood guard by the wall opposite the window. By the time Martin had set up five folding chairs around the table and arranged four vases of butter-yellow rose buds on black wrought iron flower stands in each corner, maneuvering space in the chamber was reduced to bump-and-excuse-me room.

Mrs. Hanks and Roger stepped into the chapel, squinted in the dim light, nodded to one another and to Martin, and took seats at the table in silence. Sally came next with her portable stereo. Martin helped her find a plug. She took a chair. Martin checked his watch. No Bruce. Martin tried not to fidget. After ten minutes, he said, "Let's go ahead and get started."

First, in accordance with Peter's instructions, they listened to his recording of the trio from *Der Rosenkavalier*, played on Sally's portable stereo. Three soprano voices in gentle tension moved around one another, intertwined and moved apart in a bittersweet celebration of resignation. As the voices soared and opened in a sunburst of resolution, Martin saw that this music would always be Peter's.

Then Mrs. Hanks read. "Lord, make me to know mine end, and the measure of my days, what it is; that I may know how frail I am." Sally read the translation that Peter had made for Martin of the last of Strauss's *Four Last Songs*. "The breadth and quiet of peace, the depth of the sunset . . ." Her voice quavered. "Is this then death?"

It was Roger's turn. He put on his glasses, pulled a folded paper from the breast pocket of his suit jacket, opened it, and read with slow deliberation.

Do not take rank with those poor spirits
Who neither enjoy much nor suffer much,
Because they live in the gray twilight
That knows not victory nor defeat.

Far better it is,

Even though checkered by failure,

To dare mighty things,

To win glorious triumphs.

He took off his glasses and rubbed his eyes. At first Martin thought he had finished. With the deliberateness so characteristic of him, he put his glasses on and resumed.

It is written:

Death is swallowed up in victory.

Death, where is thy sting?

Grave, where is thy victory?

Now it was Martin's turn. He had chosen Peter's translation of "The Farewell," the final song in Mahler's *Das Lied von der Erde*. The text described the last meeting between two friends at dusk by the side of a stream. The poem didn't end. It disappeared into silence. Martin's heart tightened as he read the last words, "Always . . . always . . ."

It was over.

No one moved. Then, as if by command, they rose, hugged each other, and jostled toward the vestibule.

Sally unplugged the stereo, closed it, and stood in front of Martin. "Can I talk to you a minute? Don't want to leave without saying good-bye."

"Good-bye? I hope we'll see each other once in a while."

She shook her head. "I'm going to San Francisco, to work in AIDS research. They need qualified nurses. It's not a lot of money, but it's important work."

Martin caught his breath. "I had no idea . . . Do you have any friends out there?"

"Only one. Jerry Cohen. That's who told me about it in the first place."

"His practice is here."

"Not anymore. He's going to be on the staff of San Francisco General. He'll be doing research. It's what he's always wanted."

Martin took in her words and sighed. "I hope you'll be happy in your new work."

"I'm not doing it to be happy."

She stood on tiptoe, put her arms around his neck, and kissed his cheek. "How come you had to be old enough to be my father?"

He held her for a moment. She moved away from him, picked up her stereo, and hurried out.

Martin watched her go. So like Catherine. He blinked several times and turned back to the table and the box with Peter's ashes. Roger. He glanced about. Roger was standing uncertain in the vestibule as if considering whether he could face the daylight beyond. Martin moved to his side. "Roger—"

Roger squinted toward the street. "Where I grew up and learned how things are done, we didn't mourn our dead this way. I know this was Peter's way, and I wouldn't have changed it. Now I want to do something for me. I want to go home. I want to go to Saint John of the Cross, just down the street from us. I'll ask Father Duncan to say a Mass for Peter, a Mass for the dead. That's my way."

"Will you let me know when it is, so I can come, too?" Martin asked. "And can I see you? Maybe after the Mass or some other time?"

"I don't know," Roger said. "I don't know what's going to happen next. Everything's changed. I have to start all over again. I don't know what I believe anymore." He peered into the street.

"Is Alicia all right?" Martin asked.

Roger turned back as if waking from his reverie. "No, she's not, Martin. She's going to need professional help for some time. They don't know when they'll be able to release her." He walked away, through the vestibule, down the steps, to the sidewalk, and out of sight.

Martin turned back to the deserted chapel. It was left to him to dispose of Peter's ashes. He stood for some time staring at the ugly box in the center of the table. Finally he picked it up.

Mrs. Hanks stood in his path. "You look like you could use a drink."

"I've got one more thing I have to do for Peter. I promised him I'd put his ashes in the Potomac."

She cleared her throat. "May I come with you?"

They drove through town to the 14th Street bridge, across to Virginia, along the river, past the Pentagon, past Memorial Bridge and Arlington Cemetery. Mrs. Hanks held Peter's ashes and said nothing.

"I'm surprised you wanted to come," Martin said.

"You looked like you needed a friend. And . . . Hard to explain. Sometimes in hospice work you fall in love with a patient. I fell in love with Peter. I feel privileged to be allowed to participate."

"How did you get into this kind of work?"

"Long story. I was divorced ten years ago. My two sons are fifteen and eighteen. I'd been an RN before my marriage. I didn't need a *lot* of money, so I decided to do work that was important to me."

"That wasn't so long."

"Just a little muddled."

They parked close to Roosevelt Island. A light snow was

falling. They trudged across the short footbridge, past the monumental statue of Teddy Roosevelt, and headed for the far side of the island. There, across the river from the Kennedy Center, Martin stood on the frozen bank. Somewhere, far way, cars hissed and honked. The air was wet, heavy with the scent of exhaust fumes and snow. The box in his gloved hands was weightless. An ordinary January day. He and Mrs. Hanks were ordinary people. Nothing special. No extraordinary way to say good-bye to Peter. No entourage or witnesses or mourners. Not even any tears.

He made sure he was standing in full view of the Kennedy Center, as Peter had wished. He opened the box and threw all that remained of Peter into the icy Potomac. Through the falling snow, he watched the gray ashes hit the surface, grayer still, then fade and disappear.

Now nothing was left. Peter was truly gone.

Martin raised his head, scanned the sky, and listened to the silence Peter left behind. It was odd, even eerie, that silence. Martin nodded. Peter was gone.

They returned to the car without speaking. Martin fumbled with the empty funerary box. What would he do with it? He slid it onto the back seat.

"Can I drop you somewhere?" Martin asked as he started the engine.

"Do you want that drink?"

Martin considered. "Sure. Where shall we go?"

"I have a little place in Foggy Bottom."

"That sounds obscene," he said with a frown.

"I thought it would appeal to you."

Martin drove in silence. As they neared the GW campus, he glanced at her. "You're an expert. Maybe you can advise me.

What I am going to do with the box that held Peter's ashes?"

She turned toward him. "You could save it as a reminder of Peter."

"Sounds ghoulish."

"Did you and Peter ever have a cookout?"

"No, but we went to Rock Creek Park once."

She put her hand on his shoulder. "Wait until the weather's warm and take the box to the same place you and Peter went. Find one of those stone barbecue pits. Cook something you enjoy. Before you grill it, put the box in the fire."

"Fitting way to celebrate Peter's life." He risked glancing at her. "Will you come with me?"

"Sure."

They settled at her kitchen table in a cramped apartment just off New Hampshire Avenue.

"Peter told me you like Bombay martinis," Mrs. Hanks said.

"Wonder how he knew."

She moved to the counter and mixed their drinks.

"I don't even know your first name," Martin said.

"Joanne." She brought their drinks to the table.

"*Salud*." He sipped. "Peter finally forgave himself for Johnny, a kid he infected. Died long before Peter, only five months after they had sex."

She squinted. "That's barely long enough for incubation, much less mortality. AIDS doesn't work that fast."

"Did in his case."

"Couldn't have. We know more about AIDS now. It takes at least a year to kill its victims. Someone else must have infected Johnny, long before Peter."

He glared at his drink. "My God." He fought back tears.

"Couldn't have been Peter, could it? And he suffered so because of Johnny. Jesus."

She watched him.

"No," he said. "Peter was right to grieve over Johnny. He knew he had AIDS and went ahead anyway." Martin bowed his head. "Some things are too awful to think about."

"You have a lot of grieving to do."

"Barely begun. You grieve over your patients?"

"Every one."

"I thought," Martin said, "that you professionals weren't supposed to let your feelings get in the way."

"With some of us, it's our feelings that make our work possible."

He shook his head. "I don't think I could do this kind of work for a living. I don't think I could stomach volunteering again."

"Martin, why? You were wonderful with Peter."

"Can't take the anguish."

"You really do have mourning to do, but you should feel good about what you did for Peter."

"No, I let him down. I promised him I'd be with him at the end."

"Martin," she said, "Peter didn't die alone."

"I promised. He was so scared to die."

"You stayed by Peter through his time of fear. I watched you. You were the support he used to find himself, to come to terms with death. You didn't let him down. When he was ready to die, the day he went into the hospice, he let go of you because he didn't need you any longer." She touched his sleeve. "Don't ever regret what you did for him. Take joy and pride in it."

Martin shut his eyes hard and lowered his chin to his chest.

"What am I going to do?" he whispered. "I loved him. I don't want him to be dead."

A sob broke through his defenses and escaped from his throat. She held him. His hot tears dripped on her neck. He wept, inconsolable, wishing, wishing, wishing that Peter were not dead.

◆ ◆ ◆

Sunday afternoon, Martin drove back to Roosevelt Island. He walked through the fresh snow to the far shore and gazed across the river toward the Kennedy Center, pale and massive against the seamless clouds. "We're men now," he heard Peter's voice saying. Martin smiled. It was true. Peter died a man. Martin pulled his coat collar tighter against the wind and moved along the sandy bank, stepping over the snow-lined tree roots that pushed out into the gray water. Yes, Peter was a man now. *Nice goin', Peter. You done good.*

Martin stopped and frowned. He raised his head as if listening. What had Peter said?

"Martin," he had said, "you know what? We're not no-accounts anymore. We're men now. You, too."

That's what he said.

Martin, too?

"You, too."

Martin nodded. Peter was right. So was Mort. So was Joanne. Martin had been the support Peter needed.

"Nice goin', Martin," he said aloud. "You done good."

◆ ◆ ◆

Martin met Mort Gray for dinner at Annie's the next weekend. This time, Martin insisted on paying the check.

"Healing?" Mort asked.

"I had to learn that I couldn't get over Peter's death by holding the mourning in. I've had help."

"You? The big, strong loner?"

"Mort, have you ever worked with Joanne Hanks? She's at Saint Anthony. You can chalk her up as one of the strong ones you can depend on."

"I'll remember that."

"By the way," Martin said, "I've been thinking. When I get over this, I believe I'm going to want to ask for another case."

"Glad you brought that up because I have a favor to ask. Would you be willing to take on a new patient right away?"

"Wait a minute."

"I know it's a lot to ask," Mort said, "but this is a special case. He requested you personally."

"He knows *me*?" Martin scowled at the floor. He tried to imagine how anyone could have known him. "What's his name?"

"Bruce Dushinsky."

Martin found the address—a townhouse just off O Street in Georgetown—with little trouble, but it cost him another twenty minutes to find a place to park and walk back through the fading daylight in the frozen snow. He stopped in front of the house, out of breath, his hands clammy. Why in the world was he frightened?

The house was clean and white, clapboard and dormers, the colonial door lit by two snow-covered carriage lanterns, like a nineteenth-century New England doll-house. He climbed the three steps to the paneled door and was about to knock when he saw it was ajar. He pushed it open and stepped in.

He stood in a darkened entrance hall. To his left was a narrow winding staircase. Above him hung a diminutive brass chandelier. In front of him was an open arch flanked by two sconces of glinting brass. He went through the arch.

He found himself in a sort of drawing room. The only light came from a wall of glass that looked out on a miniature garden at the back of the house. The room smelled elegant. The carpet under his feet gave no sense of a floor beneath. Drapes at the window were heavy and shining.

"Hello?" he said.

He saw a motion to his left. A young man with spiked hair the color of freshly polished copper was draped in a Chippendale chair, his head in his hands. He raised his face. His cheeks, wet with tears, shone in the gray light.

"Martin?" he said in a broken voice.

Martin watched the frightened eyes and felt a familiar hurt in his heart.

"It's me, Bruce. It's Martin."

About the Author

Tom Glenn has worked as an intelligence operative, a musician, a linguist (seven languages), a cryptologist, a government executive, a care-giver for the dying, a leadership coach, and, always, a writer. Many of his prize-winning short stories (sixteen in print) came from the better part of thirteen years he shuttled between the U.S. and Vietnam on covert intelligence assignments before being evacuated under fire when Saigon fell. His writing is haunted by his five years of work with AIDS patients, two years of helping the homeless, and seven years of caring for the dying in the hospice system. These days he is a reviewer for *The Washington Independent Review of Books* where he specializes in books on war and Vietnam. His Vietnam novel-in-stories, *Friendly Casualties*, was published in 2012 as a Kindle book on Amazon.com. His article describing the fall of Saigon and his role in it appeared in the *Baltimore Post-Examiner* in the summer of 2013. His web sites are:
http://tom-tells-tales.org
http://vietnam-tragedy.org
http://friendly-casualties.org.

Apprentice House is the country's only campus-based, student-staffed book publishing company. Directed by professors and industry professionals, it is a nonprofit activity of the Communication Department at Loyola University Maryland.

Using state-of-the-art technology and an experiential learning model of education, Apprentice House publishes books in untraditional ways. This dual responsibility as publishers and educators creates an unprecedented collaborative environment among faculty and students, while teaching tomorrow's editors, designers, and marketers.

Outside of class, progress on book projects is carried forth by the AH Book Publishing Club, a co-curricular campus organization supported by Loyola University Maryland's Office of Student Activities.

Eclectic and provocative, Apprentice House titles intend to entertain as well as spark dialogue on a variety of topics. Financial contributions to sustain the press's work are welcomed. Contributions are tax deductible to the fullest extent allowed by the IRS.

To learn more about Apprentice House books or to obtain submission guidelines, please visit www.apprenticehouse.com.

Apprentice House
Communication Department
Loyola University Maryland
4501 N. Charles Street
Baltimore, MD 21210
Ph: 410-617-5265 • Fax: 410-617-2198
info@apprenticehouse.com • www.apprenticehouse.com

CPSIA information can be obtained at www.ICGtesting.com
Printed in the USA
LVOW13s0845030414

380151LV00005B/729/P